Visual Fields

Second edition

David B. Henson

Department of Ophthalmology
University of Manchester, Manchester, UK

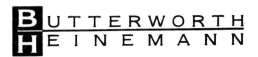

OXFORD AUCKLAND BOSTON JOHANNESBURG MELBOURNE NEW DELHI

Butterworth-Heinemann
Linacre House, Jordan Hill, Oxford OX2 8DP
225 Wildwood Avenue, Woburn, MA 01801-2041
A division of Reed Educational and Professional Publishing Ltd

A member of the Reed Elsevier plc group

First published 1993
Second edition published 2000

British Library Cataloguing in Publication Data

Henson, David B.
  Visual Fields. – 2nd ed.
  1. Visual Fields   2. Perimetry   3. Eye – Diseases – Diagnosis
  I. Title
  617.7'15

Library of Congress Cataloguing in Publication Data

Henson, David B.
  Visual Fields/David B. Henson. – 2nd ed.
  p. cm.
  Originally published: Oxford; New York, 1993 in series (Oxford medical publications).
  Includes bibliographical references and index.
  ISBN 0 7506 4173 8
  1. Perimetry.   2. Visual fields.   I. Title.

  RE79.P4 H45
  617.7'15–dc21   00–031206

ISBN 0 7506 4173 8

Typeset by David Gregson Associates, Beccles, Suffolk
Printed and bound in Great Britain, by Martins the Printers, Berwick upon Tweed

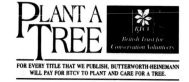

Contents

1 Introduction

Welcome to 'Visual Fields', a book designed to give you a comprehensive overview of the clinical aspects of visual field testing.

Included in this text are practical details on how to measure the visual field as well as theoretical details to help the clinician understand the basis of perimetry and get to grips with all the different techniques that are currently being used.

Like almost every other discipline, perimetry has developed its own language. While this helps perimetrists to communicate with each other it can, for the new student, lead to both confusion and misunderstanding. In an attempt to help the student overcome this problem, a Glossary of Terms is provided at the end of the book.

The remainder of this chapter covers some of the basic aspects of visual fields. It includes a definition of the visual field and introduces the reader to the frequently used units of measurement and some of the conventions that have been adopted by perimetrists. As it is primarily designed for the new student of perimetry, those readers who are already familiar with these topics might wish to go on to the next chapter or to a chapter whose subject is of particular interest.

DEFINITION OF THE VISUAL FIELD

If for a moment you can imagine yourself sitting in a room looking at a large wall, then the visual field is the area of wall that can be seen without moving your eyes or head. If you actually try this then you will probably find that no matter how large the wall is you can always see at least one edge/corner. This is because the visual field extends beyond 90 degrees in the temporal

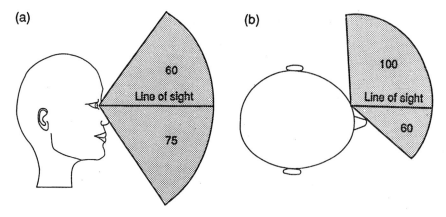

Fig. 1.1 *Vertical and horizontal extent of the normal visual field.*

direction and it is impossible to map its full extent on a flat surface.

Tate and Lynn (1977) defined the visual field as 'all the space that one eye can see at any given instant'. Tate and Lynn use the term 'space' to highlight the fact that the eye is looking at a three-dimensional volume of space rather than a two-dimensional area.

If for the moment we consider the eye to be like a camera, the retina being represented by the film, then we can appreciate that if we were to take a photograph of a three-dimensional scene we would end up with a two-dimensional photograph. The camera has converted the three-dimensional scene into a two-dimensional photograph. The retina of each eye works in the same way; it converts the three-dimensional space into two dimensions. Perimetrists, therefore, normally represent the visual field in two dimensions and talk about the 'area' of the visual field rather than its 'volume'. It is interesting to note, however, that the visual system can retrieve a certain amount of three-dimensional information by combining the slightly different images from the two eyes.

Perimetry is defined simply as the study of the visual field and a perimeter is an instrument designed for perimetry. While any instrument designed to measure the visual field could be called a perimeter, most clinicians reserve the term to describe those instruments that are capable of measuring the whole extent of the visual field. Instruments that only measure the central fields are variously described as central field analysers, tangent screens etc.

EXTENT OF THE NORMAL VISUAL FIELD
The normal extent of the visual field, for a bright stimulus is:

60 degrees UP
75 degrees DOWN
100 degrees TEMPORAL
60 degrees NASAL

(see Figure 1.1).

The bridge of the nose influences the nasal extent. Patients with prominent bridges will have a reduced nasal field. The superior extent is also affected by facial contours. Patients with deep-set eyes or prominent brows will have a restricted superior field.

The effect of facial contours can, to some extent, be overcome during perimetry by getting the patient to turn his or her head. For example, in an individual with a prominent brow the full extent of the field can be measured by getting the patient to lift the chin slightly, turning the face upwards (see Figure 1.2). You can easily demonstrate this effect to yourself. Again look at a point on a wall directly in front of you and then, while continuing to fixate the same point, move your head up and down in a nodding fashion. You will notice that when your face is turned down you can only see a small part of the wall above your fixation point. As you turn your face up, then you will gradually increase the superior extent of your visual field.

With both eyes open the visual field has a horizontal extent of approximately 200 degrees (100 degrees

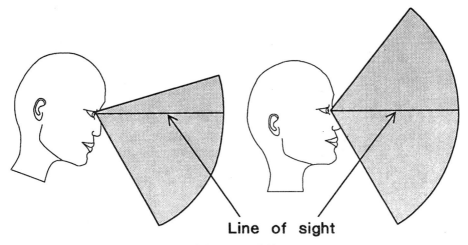

Line of sight

Fig. 1.2 *Influence of head posture upon the extent of the superior field.*

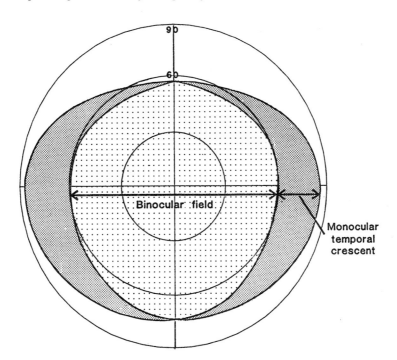

Fig. 1.3 *Extent of the binocular visual field.*

temporal for each eye) while the vertical extent obviously remains the same (see Figure 1.3).

The binocular visual field, that is, the region where both eyes can see the stimulus, extends for approximately 60 degrees on either side of the vertical midline, 60 degrees up and 75 degrees down. The inferior extent of the binocular field is, however, affected by the nose.

ISLAND OF VISION

The sensitivity of the eye is not constant across the whole of the visual field but varies in a rather complicated way with eccentricity, adaptation level and the nature of the test stimulus (see Chapter 2 for more details). As a means of representing the different sensitivities at different regions, the visual field is often described as an island, a concept attributed to

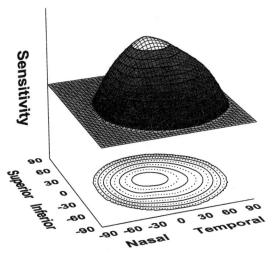

Fig. 1.4   *The island of vision.*

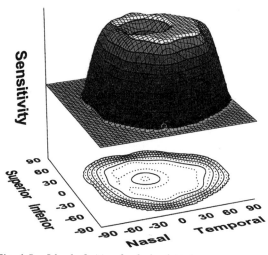

Fig. 1.5   *Island of vision for dark-adapted eye.*

Traquair, who described the visual field as an 'Island of vision in a sea of darkness' (see Figure 1.4).

The height, or elevation, of the island represents the sensitivity of the eye. Stimuli whose parameters place them above the island are too weak to be seen. Those that fall outside of the island (over the sea) are outside of the field of view (e.g. behind your head) and cannot be seen no matter how bright they are made. Only stimuli whose parameters place them within the island of vision can be seen.

Just as geographers use contour lines to represent the height of an island on a map so perimetrists use isopters to represent the sensitivity of the eye on a field chart. A contour line is a line joining points of equal height above sea level. An isopter is a line joining points of equal sensitivity (see Figure 1.4).

There is, at least, one major difference between geographical islands and islands of vision. Geographical islands are fixed. They do not change significantly from one minute to the next. The island of vision changes with the state of adaptation. When the eye is light-adapted it will appear as a relatively low-lying island with a peak at its centre, the fovea. When the eye is dark-adapted the island will be much higher (more sensitive) and because of the distribution of rods and cones will have a crater at its centre (see Figure 1.5). This sensitivity to external factors is one reason why perimeters, if they are to be used to compare one result with another, must be able to keep external factors, such as background intensity, under control.

PRESENTATION OF VISUAL FIELD DATA

Graphically presenting the data from a visual field examination or mapping the visual field, a term derived from Traquair's island of vision concept, can take many different forms. The simplest of these is the isopter map (see Figure 1.6). This type of map is derived from a technique in which a stimulus of fixed strength is moved from outside of the island (where it cannot be seen) towards its centre until it is seen, i.e. first touches the surface. This point represents the limit of the field for that particular stimulus. By repeating this measurement along different approach directions a

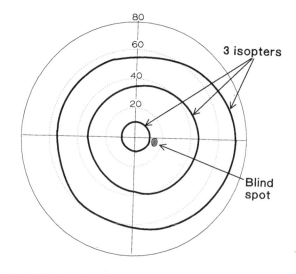

Fig. 1.6   *A series of isopters.*

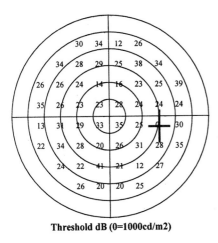

Fig. 1.7 *Visual field chart giving the eye's sensitivity at a series of different retinal locations.*

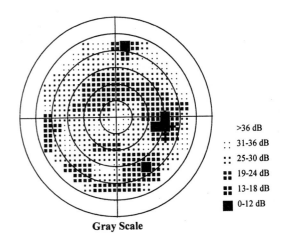

Fig. 1.8 *Grey scale representation of the eye's sensitivity.*

series of points of equal sensitivity can be obtained which when joined together form an isopter. A different stimulus, one that is either weaker or stronger than the first, can then be used to produce another isopter. Using the analogy of an island, it is a bit like flying toward the island at a fixed height above sea level and seeing where you first make contact!

An alternative form of mapping the visual field is to choose a location over the island and then gradually increase the strength of the stimulus until it is seen. Again, using the analogy of an island, it is like hovering in a helicopter above the island and then gradually coming down until you land. Using this technique at a series of different locations it is again possible to end up with some idea of the island's contour. Continuing with the analogy of mapping, it is like having a series of different spot heights. With enough spot height measurements it is possible to extrapolate where the isopters should go and hence produce an isopter diagram of the island. It is, however, more usual to represent data collected in this way as a series of spot heights (see Figure 1.7). To improve the appearance of the results extrapolated measures are often used to fill in the spaces between actual measurements, and to represent sensitivity with grey scale symbols (see Figure 1.8).

WHY DO WE MEASURE THE VISUAL FIELD?

There are many different ways in which a patient's vision can be assessed. We can measure visual acuity,

the extent of the visual field, the rate at which the eye adapts to the dark or the small electrical potentials that arise from the eye and cortex, to name but a few. Perimetry is just one of a whole series of different techniques at the clinician's disposal to assess visual function. Each technique has its own merits and shortcomings.

One of the merits of perimetry is that it is one of the few techniques that evaluate the peripheral retina and the neural pathways responsible for relaying information from the peripheral retinal to the higher centres of the brain. As there are certain conditions which primarily, or only, affect the peripheral retina or its pathways, perimetry clearly has a very important role to play in their detection.

Perimetry has another advantage in that it is a direct measure of visual function. Other tests, such as a measurement of the intraocular pressure, may lead us to think that visual function is being damaged but are not a measure of that damage. Repeat perimetric examinations are particularly valuable for monitoring the progression of, or recovery from, conditions affecting the peripheral retina and pathways. In this capacity they are particularly good at monitoring the efficacy of a given form of treatment. Remember treatment of the eye is primarily aimed at either maintaining or regaining visual function, which is exactly what perimetrists are measuring.

Perimetry can aid differential diagnosis. Certain conditions, such as glaucoma and chiasmal compression, give characteristic patterns of visual field loss.

Finally, perimetry is a simple, non-invasive technique that can be applied to almost all ages with no discomfort or adverse reactions, although it should be added that, on occasions, it can be a little tedious.

UNITS OF MEASUREMENT
Position of stimulus
By convention, the position of a stimulus within the visual field is described in terms of its eccentricity, how far it is away from the fixation point (measured in degrees), and the meridian along which the target lies. The horizontal corresponds to the 0 and 180 degree meridian and the vertical to the 90 and 270 degrees meridian (see Figure 1.9). It is also common for the eccentricity of the target to be described in general descriptive terms, such as peripheral, central, mid-periphery, centrocecal etc., and for the radial position to be specified according to which quadrant it falls in, i.e. superior temporal, superior nasal, inferior nasal and inferior temporal.

Size of stimulus
The specification of stimulus size varies with the type of examination. Most instruments now specify the size in terms of the angle subtended at the eye, e.g. a target subtends 30 minutes of arc (0.5 degrees) (see Figure 1.10). There are, however, two major exceptions to this. With bowl type perimeters it is common to

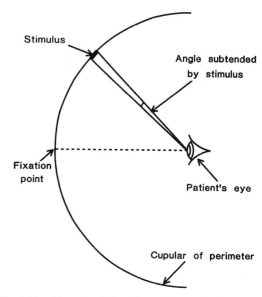

Fig. 1.10 *Normal technique for specifying stimulus size.*

refer to the stimulus size as being equivalent to one of those used in the Goldmann bowl perimeter. Goldmann's bowl perimeter has six different target sizes, labelled 0, I, II, III, IV and V. The nominal size and angle subtended by these stimuli are given in Table 1.1. The other exception is when a tangent screen is used. A tangent screen is a large flat cloth or screen often attached to a wall. It is common with this type of instrument to refer to the size of the target in millimetres, in which case the number refers to the target's diameter. To calculate the angle subtended by the target it is necessary to know the testing distance and this is usually incorporated into the stimulus specification which is given as a fraction, the numerator being the target size and the denominator the testing distance. For example a target specification of

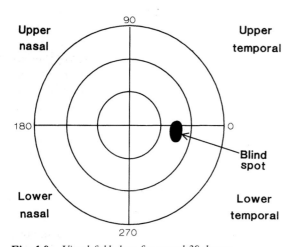

Fig. 1.9 *Visual field chart for central 30 degrees*

Table 1.1 Size of stimuli used by Goldmann

Goldmann size	Nominal size (mm^2)	Angular subtence (min of arc)
0	0.0625	3.78
I	0.25	7.68
II	1.0	15.36
III	4.0	30.71
IV	16	61.3
V	64	122.56

2/1000 means that the target's diameter is 2 mm and the testing distance is 1000 mm (1 m).

Stimulus intensity

Stimulus intensity specifications are rather more complicated and there are three main concepts the reader needs to grasp.

The first is that perimetrists rarely talk about the 'intensity' of a stimulus; they prefer to talk about the eye's 'sensitivity'. Sensitivity scales are the inverse of intensity scales. As the sensitivity of the eye goes up it is capable of seeing dimmer and dimmer stimuli.

To make things even more confusing, it is also common for perimetrists to talk about the eye's threshold. The eye's threshold is normally given in terms of stimulus intensity. In other words, as the threshold goes down the stimulus intensity goes down and the eye's sensitivity goes up.

I fear some of you may be beginning to question whether you have chosen to study the right subject! Take comfort in the fact that even those who have been studying perimetry for many years still occasionally get confused when it comes to talking about sensitivity and thresholds.

The second concept is that stimulus and background intensities are normally specified in luminance units. Now, luminance measures tell you how bright something appears, they are different from units of illumination which tell you how much light is falling on a surface. As an example, suppose for the moment there are two walls, one is painted black and the other white, with the same amount of light falling on each. If we measure the luminance of the walls, that is the amount of light reflected off the wall, then we would find that the black wall has a very low luminance in comparison to the white one. Yet their illumination, that is the amount of light falling upon the walls, is the same. In perimetry we are interested in stating how bright the background and stimuli appear to the eye and hence we use luminance units. Having said that, there are, as always, a few exceptions. Some of the older instruments, such as the Bjerrum screen, are normally set up with a fixed level of illumination.

The units for luminance are candelas per square metre (cd/m^2) and apostilbs (asb) (1 cd/m^2 = 3.14 asb).

The third concept concerns stimulus and background intensities, and it is possibly the most

Table 1.2 Relationship between decibel and logarithmic attenuation scales and the intensity of a perimetric stimulus

Decibel scale	Log scale	Intensity luminance units
0	0	1000
10	1	100
20	2	10
30	3	1
40	4	0.1

difficult one for the new student to grasp. Stimulus and background intensities are normally presented on logarithmic rather than linear scales. Now the important thing to remember about logarithmic scales is that for each unit change in the log scale there is a 10-fold change in intensity (or sensitivity) (see Table 1.2).

It is also fairly common for the results of an examination to be specified in decibels (dB) rather than log units. In perimetry a decibel scale is simply a logarithmic scale where 10 decibels equals 1 log unit (see Table 1.2).

One of the effects of using a log/decibel scale is to compress the axis. For example, if the luminance of the eye changes from 1000 cd/m^2 to 10 units (a 100-fold change) we can see from Table 1.2 that when plotted on a log scale it would only change from 0 to 2. Another effect is to give greater significance to the lower end of the scale.

So why do we want to compress the axis and give more significance to the lower end of the scale? Well, there are two reasons. The first is that the eye can operate over a very large range of intensities, something in the order of 10 000 000 fold. If we were to use a linear scale that went from 0 to 10 000 000 then small, but significant, changes in sensitivity at the lower end of the scale would not be discernible. The second, and more important reason, is that the eye, as well as the other senses, appears to operate on something close to a logarithmic scale. If asked to make a judgement as to how much brighter one light is in comparison to another, responses appear to follow a logarithmic, rather than linear, scale.

Another confusing aspect about the specification of stimulus and background intensities is that many of the new field analysers refer to the intensity of a stimulus simply in terms of its decibel or logarithmic value.

Now, those of you with any background in mathematics will immediately realize that decibels and log units are NOT a measure of luminance. So, when the printout from one of these instruments tells you that the sensitivity of a given test location is 32 dB what does this mean? Well, somewhere on the printout, or in the instrument's manual, you should be able to find a statement that tells you what 0 dB corresponds to in luminance units. For example, you may find it says that at 0 dB the stimulus intensity is 1000 asb, or at 0 dB the stimulus intensity is 300 cd/m^2. Values above 0 then refer to an attenuation of this intensity. Once you know what the 0 level corresponds to you can quickly calculate what the stimulus intensity is in luminance units (see Table 1.2). In reality, perimetrists simply talk about defects in terms of decibels, e.g. the patient has a 10 dB loss in the nasal field.

Now some of you must be thinking that this is an awfully complicated way of doing things. Why not just give the value in luminance units? Well there are two advantages to following the convention. The first is that the log and decibel scales go up as the intensity scale goes down. Thus the log/decibel attenuation scales are akin to sensitivity scales. As the eye's sensitivity goes up so too do the log/decibel values and there is, I think, some logic in having high numbers represent high sensitivities rather than the reverse. The second advantage is that the eye, as mentioned before, appears to work in log/decibel units and it is better, therefore, to represent losses etc. in log/decibel units rather than luminance units.

CONCLUDING REMARKS

By now you should have gained a sufficient knowledge of the basic concepts of perimetry to get you through the rest of this text. Don't forget that if you come across a word that you don't understand, try looking it up in the Glossary. If you cannot find it there or want another definition try one of the dictionaries of visual science, such as Cline *et al.* (1980) or Millodot (1997).

REFERENCES

Cline D., Hofstetter H.W. and Griffin J.R. (1980) *Dictionary of Visual Science*. Chilton, Pennsylvania.

Millodot M. (1997) *Dictionary of Optometry and Visual Science*, 4th edn. Butterworth–Heinemann, Oxford.

Tate G.W. and Lynn J.R. (1977) *Principles of Quantitative Perimetry*. Grune and Stratton, New York.

2 Psychophysics

INTRODUCTION

The introductory chapter, Chapter 1, briefly mentioned how the eye's sensitivity varies with different parameters such as stimulus intensity, stimulus size, background intensity etc. It did not, however, mention all the parameters that can affect the results of a visual field examination or establish what the relationships are between different stimulus parameters.

In this chapter these parameters will be studied in more detail. We are going to investigate what the exact relationships are between the threshold of a stimulus and its size, its presentation time, its position etc.

The study of the interrelationships between the physical parameters of a stimulus and its perception is known as psychophysics. It is a subject that has been studied at great length by many researchers and there are several textbooks devoted solely to the subject. In comparison to these, this chapter will offer a quick summary of those parameters that are particularly relevant to the clinical testing of the visual field.

These include:

1. Background luminance and adaptation time.
2. Stimulus size.
3. Stimulus presentation time.
4. Stimulus speed of movement.
5. Colour of stimulus.
6. Psychological factors, the frequency-of-seeing curve.

BACKGROUND LUMINANCE
Introduction
The background luminance is important in visual field testing because:

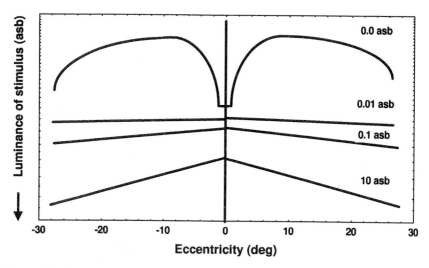

Fig. 2.1 *Sensitivity profiles for four different background intensity levels.*

(i) it controls the sensitivity profile, i.e. how the sensitivity changes with eccentricity;

(ii) it controls the length of time that the patient needs to adapt before the start of an examination.

Background luminance and the sensitivity profile

Figure 2.1 gives sensitivity profiles for a number of different background luminances. At high, photopic, luminances the profile has a peak at the centre of the field, the fovea. At lower background intensities, the mesopic level, the profile is almost flat, showing very little change in sensitivity with eccentricity. At very low luminance levels the peak sensitivity occurs at an eccentricity of around 15 degrees, falling off at the fovea and towards the periphery. It is important to stress that the sensitivity of the whole retina increases with reduced background intensities. The change in profile results from the peripheral sensitivity increasing at a faster rate than the foveal sensitivity.

Background luminance and adaptation time

We are all aware of what happens when we walk into a dimly lit cinema. While initially it is very difficult to see any detail, after a few moments our eyes get used to the dark and we can begin to recognize things. Our eyes have adapted to the new level of illumination and become more sensitive. When we go back outside the reverse happens. We are initially dazzled by the bright sunlight but soon get used to it. Our eyes light-adapt and become less sensitive. In order to get accurate results from a visual field examination it is important that we wait for the eyes' sensitivity to stabilize – for the eyes to adapt to the background luminance. If we fail to do this then the results are likely to be more variable, particularly during the early stages of the examination.

The time necessary for adaptation to be complete is dependent upon:

(a) The background level.
(b) The prior state of adaptation.
(c) The period of pre-adaptation.

Figure 2.2 demonstrates how the eye's threshold reduces with time when it is placed in the dark after being pre-adapted to four different luminance levels. Examination of this figure shows that it can take over 30 minutes for the eye's threshold to stabilize after it has been pre-adapted to a particularly high luminance level.

The relationship between the period of pre-adaptation and subsequent adaptation is given in Figure 2.3. Note that the longer the pre-adapting period, the longer it takes for the eye's sensitivity to stabilize. These two factors, intensity and duration of pre-adapting light, are simply a reflection of how the rate of adaptation is dependent upon the total amount of retinal bleaching.

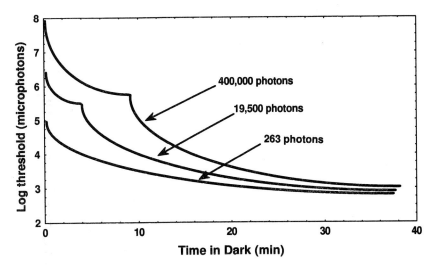

Fig. 2.2 *Adaptation curves for three different pre-adapting luminance levels.*

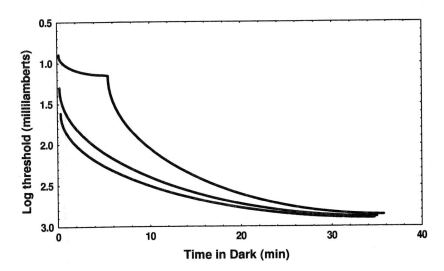

Fig. 2.3 *Adaptation curves for three different pre-adaptation times, adapting luminance 333 millilamberts.*

Of particular relevance to perimetry is the time required for the eye's sensitivity to stabilize to the background intensities used in most modern perimeters (see Figure 2.4), rather than the time necessary for it to adapt to complete darkness. Unfortunately, there seems to be a relative paucity of published data on this subject. Figure 2.5 gives some data, which demonstrate that the time necessary for the eye's sensitivity to stabilize is shorter for the higher background intensities. These data were obtained after the eyes were adapted to a luminance that is consider-

ably higher than that experienced in a normal room and, therefore, overestimate adaptation times for patients who have been sitting in the waiting room prior to their visual field examination.

It is important to stress that a fundus examination can dramatically affect adaptation time. The retinal illumination produced by both direct and indirect ophthalmoscopes (and most other forms of fundus examination) is very high and will cause a considerable amount of retinal bleaching (see Table 2.1). It would, therefore, be better to arrange for the visual field

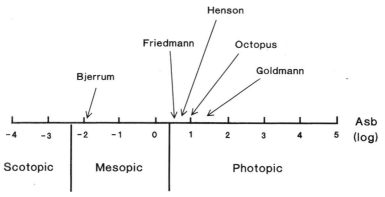

Fig. 2.4 *Background intensity levels used in several visual field instruments.*

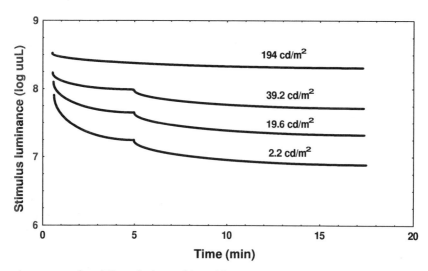

Fig. 2.5 *Adaptation curves to four different background intensities.*

Table 2.1 Retinal illumination produced by different ophthalmic instruments

Types of examination	Retinal illumination (mW/cm^2)
Direct ophthalmoscopy	29
Indirect ophthalmoscopy	70
Slit lamp	200

Source: Data taken from Calkins *et al.* (1980)

examination to precede any fundus examination or at least ensure that ophthalmoscopy does not immediately precede the visual field examination.

The problem of adaptation is further complicated by a relationship between adaptation and eccentricity.

Different regions of the retina, generally those of potentially greater sensitivity, take longer to fully adapt than do others.

What has been said thus far assumes that the whole eye is exposed to the same intensity levels, which is the usual case in perimetry. It is, however, possible to have local adaptation where a specific region of the retina is adapted to a different level than other regions. A bright spot of light can result in a locally adapted area where the sensitivity of the eye is below that of neighbouring regions. This type of situation can occur during perimetry if the fixation target is bright in comparison to the rest of the field. In such situations the area surrounding the fixation target may appear to have a depressed sensitivity.

Factors influencing the choice of background luminance

In deciding an appropriate background luminance for perimetry there are several questions that should be asked.

Are the visual field defects we are looking for dependent upon background luminance?

Clearly, if the visual field defect is more pronounced at certain background luminances then these should be used. Of course, the question is complicated by the fact that while certain pathological conditions may very well show a relationship between their extent of loss and the background luminance other pathologies will not. For example, the field loss seen in retinitis pigmentosa is known to be more apparent at low luminance levels. On the other hand, glaucomatous defects have been reported to be relatively independent of background luminance.

Is there any advantage in having a particular sensitivity profile?

In kinetic perimetry, when we are moving the stimulus towards the fovea and recording when it first becomes visible, the amount of variability in the isopter location is dependent upon the sensitivity profile. Consider, for a moment, Figure 2.6. In this figure there are two sensitivity profiles, one steep and the other shallow.

If a stimulus is brought from the periphery to the centre of the field then it will contact the sensitivity profile at a given eccentricity. This is the point at which the stimulus first becomes visible and the point that would mark the isopter position. So far so good. The problem is that the sensitivity of the eye does not remain constant, it fluctuates over a small range of values (see *Psychological factors: the frequency-of-seeing curve*, p. 19). This fluctuation is equivalent to the island of vision bobbing up and down over a small range of values, as is shown by the shaded area in Figure 2.6. Now if the sensitivity profile is shallow this fluctuation will result in much larger shifts in the position of the isopter than will occur when the sensitivity profile is steep. Isopter positions will, therefore, be more variable when the sensitivity profile is shallow, as occurs at mesopic background luminance levels. This is, in fact, one of the reasons Goldmann chose to use a relatively high background luminance in his bowl perimeter. This point concerning background luminance is, of course, only relevant to kinetic visual field testing. With static techniques the accuracy of the result is not dependent on the sensitivity profile.

Is it possible to maintain certain background luminances more easily than others?

The simple answer to this question is 'yes'. The

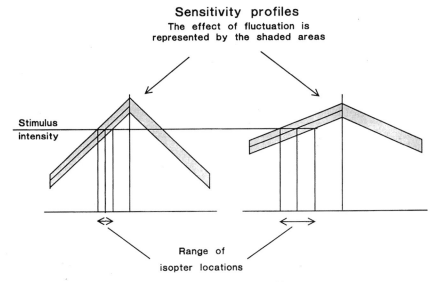

Sensitivity profiles
The effect of fluctuation is represented by the shaded areas

Stimulus intensity

Range of isopter locations

Fig. 2.6 *The effect of fluctuation on isopter position for two different profiles.*

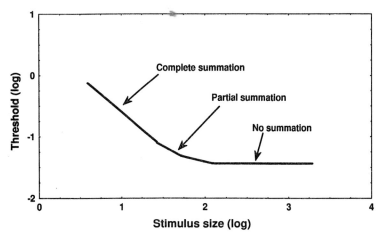

Fig. 2.7 *The relationship between stimulus size and threshold.*

majority of visual field instruments are, at least partially, sensitive to ambient illumination and need to be operated in a room in which the ambient illumination can be controlled. Now anyone who has worked in a clinical environment will appreciate that it is very difficult to have absolute control over the ambient illumination – doors are often being opened and closed etc. It is, therefore, better to choose a background luminance that is relatively insensitive to small fluctuations in the room's ambient illumination, i.e. one that is fairly bright.

Is the variability of the patient's responses dependent upon the background luminance?

If variability were dependent upon background luminance then clearly it would be better to choose an intensity at which the variability is at a minimum. This particular point was investigated by Greve (1973), who concluded that there is no difference in the variability of results at mesopic and photopic adaptation levels.

Currently used background luminance levels

Having attempted to answer to all these questions, what then are the luminance levels that have been chosen for the background of modern perimeters? Figure 2.4 shows a luminance scale upon which the values for many instruments are marked. A large number of instruments have chosen to use the Goldmann level of $10 \, \text{cd/m}^2$. Others have tended

to use lower intensity levels where the sensitivity profile is flatter. All instruments, with the exception of the Bjerrum screen, use photopic levels where adaptation times are relatively short. Clearly, those instruments that use higher background luminances have the advantage of shorter adaptation times and a reduced sensitivity to fluctuations in ambient illumination.

STIMULUS SIZE
Introduction

Within a certain range of stimulus sizes there is a simple relationship between the size of a stimulus and its threshold. The larger the size, the lower the threshold (see Figure 2.7). This relationship, which is known as spatial summation, is due to a convergence of neural elements within the retina. A peripheral retinal ganglion cell receives input from a large number of receptors whose receptive fields are spread over a small area of the visual field. The ganglion cell will signal a response when the combined input reaches a threshold value. In other words, it will respond either when a few cells are strongly stimulated, a small bright stimulus, or when a larger number of cells are weakly stimulated, a large dim stimulus.

Ricco's and Pieron's laws

For small stimuli, summation is practically complete and can be represented by the equation:

$$\text{Log luminance} + \text{log area} = \text{Constant}$$

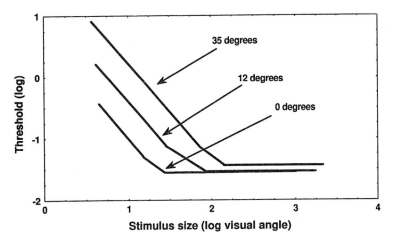

Fig. 2.8 *The relationship between stimulus size and threshold at different retinal eccentricities in the light-adapted eye.*

or
$$\text{Luminance} \times \text{Area} = \text{Constant}$$

This is known as Ricco's law. Beyond the size where summation is complete lies a range of stimulus sizes where summation still operates but no longer obeys Ricco's law, i.e. there is partial summation. This can be represented by the more general form of the equation:

$$\text{Log luminance} + K(\log \text{area}) = \text{Constant}$$

or
$$\text{Luminance} \times (\text{Area})^{\wedge}K = \text{Constant}$$

where K is a constant known as the summation coefficient whose value is always less than 1 and tends to 0 as the area of the stimulus extends beyond the summation area. This equation is known as Pieron's law.

V. pero law

The effects of adaptation and eccentricity upon spatial summation

The extent of spatial summation varies with both eccentricity and adaptation level. In the dark-adapted eye the zone of complete summation varies from less than 30 minutes of arc at the fovea to around 60 minutes of arc at the periphery.

In the light-adapted eye the zone of complete summation is smaller and the relationship with eccentricity linear (see Figure 2.8) (Wilson, 1970; Lie, 1980).

One of the effects of the summation area varying with eccentricity is that the sensitivity profile also changes with stimulus size (see Figure 2.9) (Lie, 1980).

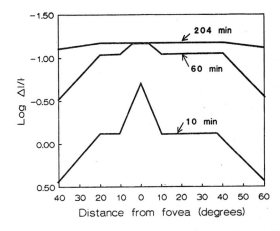

Fig. 2.9 *The effect of stimulus size on the sensitivity profile.*

Spatial summation and perimetry

Spatial summation is very important to the perimetrist as it is the basis upon which size and intensity can be substituted for each other in instruments such as the Goldmann bowl perimeter and the Bjerrum screen.

When Goldmann first developed his perimeter he raised the question of possible changes in retinal summation with pathological conditions. He suggested that one of the first functions to be damaged by retinal pathology might be spatial summation. He, therefore, decided to use stimuli whose sizes changed by steps, which were equivalent to intensity changes of 5 dB. Altering the size by one step and the intensity by 5 dB in the opposite direction should, if summation is normal, result in an identical isopter. By and large this is exactly what you find with the Goldmann perimeter, although there are limitations with respect to the size of the stimuli and the areas of the retina over which the relationship is valid.

This subject was investigated at great length by Dubois-Poulson and Magis (1959), who used the term 'photometric disharmony' to describe the breakdown of the normal relationship between the size and intensity of perimetric stimuli. They defined disharmony as an isopter difference of 10 degrees or more when equivalent stimuli are used on the Goldmann perimeter (Greve, 1973). Although photometric disharmony has been reported to exist in a large number of different pathologies there is a great deal of individual variability. It is, therefore, unwise to make any conclusions solely on the basis of disharmony.

Before leaving the subject of spatial summation there is one final point that needs to be made. If an eye with an uncorrected refractive error views the stimulus, then this effectively produces a larger and dimmer stimulus on the retina. Depending upon the initial size of the stimulus and the extent of the blur this can have a significant effect upon the patient's measured sensitivity. More details on the effects of defocus can be found in Chapter 5 which examines 'parameters affecting visual field results'.

STIMULUS PRESENTATION TIME
Introduction
The visual system temporally sums signals that fall within what is known as 'the critical duration of vision'. In other words, a stimulus will appear brighter the longer it is exposed until its exposure time exceeds the critical duration, which in the human eye is in the order of 100 msec.

Up to the critical duration time summation is almost perfect. If you double the exposure time of a stimulus which is at threshold and then reduce its intensity until it is back at threshold level, then you will find that this new level is approximately half that of the original one. In other words, the product of luminance and time is a constant when the stimulus is at threshold.

Bloch's law
The relationship between luminance and duration is known as Bloch's law, which simply states that up to the critical duration time:

$$\text{Luminance} \times \text{duration} = \text{Constant}$$

When the duration of a stimulus exceeds the critical duration, the effect of a test light becomes independent of its duration.

The effects of stimulus size, background luminance and retinal location upon the critical duration
Temporal summation and the critical duration vary according to:

(a) Stimulus size.
(b) Background luminance.
(c) Retinal location.

Figure 2.10 demonstrates how it changes with stimulus size: the larger the stimulus, the shorter the critical duration. Figure 2.11 demonstrates how it changes with background luminance: the higher the background luminance, the shorter the critical duration. Both these sets of results are for foveal fixation. For peripheral targets, the critical duration is a little longer.

Temporal summation and perimetry
What relevance does temporal summation have to visual field testing? The first, and obvious, point to make is that when presentation times are below the critical duration then it is essential that both the luminance and the duration of the stimulus be defined. If presentation times exceed the critical duration then it is only necessary to specify the stimulus luminance as detection becomes solely dependent upon this. In clinical examinations stimuli are, therefore, normally presented for longer than the critical duration as this excludes stimulus duration as a variable.

There is another point that needs to be considered with respect to presentation times. The sudden appearance of a peripheral light would normally result in the patient looking towards the stimulus, the orientating reflex. Even though the patient is instructed to try to suppress this reflex during the examination, inevitably there are going to be some occasions where the patient looks towards the stimulus. The normal saccadic reaction time, that is the time between the presentation of a stimulus and

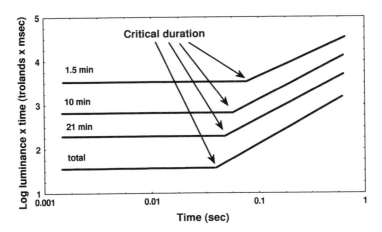

Fig. 2.10 *The critical duration for four different sizes of stimulus.*

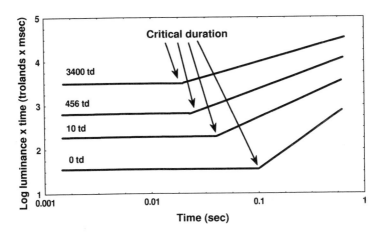

Fig. 2.11 *The critical duration for four different background luminances.*

the first eye movement, is approximately 250 msec. To stop these movements from influencing the results, the presentation time should be kept below the normal saccadic reaction time, i.e. by the time the patient starts to move their eyes the stimulus has already been turned off.

Taking all this into account it would appear that the ideal presentation time would lie between 100 and 250 msec, i.e. longer than the critical duration and shorter than the saccadic reaction time. The majority of static perimeters use presentation times of 200 msec.

STIMULUS SPEED OF MOVEMENT
Introduction
The speed of stimulus movement is, clearly, only

relevant to kinetic techniques of investigation, and there are two points concerning the speed of movement which are important to the perimetrist. The first concerns the reaction times of the patient and perimetrist. If the stimulus is moving relatively fast then it can travel quite a distance between being detected by the patient and recorded by the perimetrist. In such instances the recorded isopters will be closer to the fixation point and the island of vision will appear to have sunk a little. If the perimetrist was plotting the extent of a scotoma, moving from the non-seeing to the seeing, then the size of the scotoma will appear larger.

The second point concerns the patient's level of attention. It has already been mentioned, and will be mentioned in more detail later on, that a patient's sensitivity changes with time. It is as if the island of vision is bobbing up and down. There is some evidence to show that this fluctuation can be reduced by giving patients some form of signal, or warning, a second or so before the stimulus is presented. This signal, which in static perimetry is often an auditory tone, 'sets' the patient, makes them pay attention. If nothing happens within the next second or so, then they go back to their old habit of bobbing up and down.

If we consider what happens in kinetic testing then we can see how the speed of movement may influence the level of set and subsequent accuracy of results. In this form of perimetry the patient is set by the verbal instructions of the perimetrist. For example, the perimetrist may say, 'I'm going to bring the stimulus in, tell me when you can first see it'. This sets the patient. If the stimulus is now moved, very slowly, towards the fixation point, then by the time it reaches the point at which the patient can see it any level of set will have totally disappeared and there will be a tendency for the results to become more variable. Most experienced perimetrists are well aware of this problem and adjust the speed of stimulus movement and the starting position to produce a response within the ideal period.

This is one reason why an experienced perimetrist obtains more reliable results with kinetic instruments, such as the Goldmann bowl perimeter.

Recommended speed of movement

So what is the recommended speed of movement for a kinetic stimulus? Goldmann (1945) suggests 5 degrees per second in the peripheral field. Others have suggested speeds of 2 deg/sec.

As yet there is no definitive research on the optimal speed of movement, and even if there were it would most likely vary from one patient to another.

COLOUR OF STIMULUS
Introduction
Conventional perimetry uses a white stimulus on a white background, but what happens if we change the colour of the stimulus and/or background? Are there any benefits likely to accrue from the use of coloured stimuli and if so how might these best be incorporated into routine investigative techniques?

The sensation of colour is mediated by the retinal cones, which are classified into three groups according to which wavelengths of light they are most sensitive to. There are those that respond best to short wavelength light, the blue cones, those that respond best to the middle wavelengths, the green cones, and those that respond best to the long wavelengths, the red cones (see Figure 2.12).

In the peripheral field the density of cones per unit angle is much lower than it is at the fovea, and although there is good evidence to suggest that the rods contribute to the peripheral perception of colour, the peripheral colour sense is much worse than that of the fovea.

Chromatic and achromatic thresholds

There are two ways in which the patient can be asked to respond to a coloured stimulus:

(1) The patient can be asked to report when he or she first sees the stimulus – the achromatic threshold.
(2) The patient can be asked to report when he or she can first identify the colour of the stimulus – the chromatic threshold.

The two are not the same. Patients can usually report being able to see a stimulus before being able to identify its colour. The difference between the two thresholds is known as the chromatic interval, which, of course, varies with a whole host of factors such as

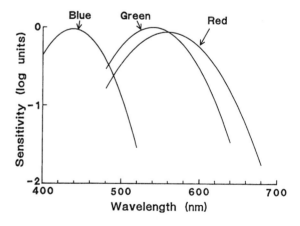

Fig. 2.12 *Spectral sensitivity curves for the blue, green and red cones. The red curve has been displaced vertically to aid visualization.*

eccentricity and state of adaptation. It is also of interest to note that the variability of achromatic thresholds is similar to that of conventional white stimuli while the variability of chromatic thresholds is much greater. It is far more difficult for patients to identify the intensity at which they can just recognize the colour of a stimulus than it is for them to identify the intensity at which they can just see a stimulus.

It is also important to realize that coloured stimuli are occasionally used as an alternative means of reducing the intensity of a stimulus. On the Bjerrum screen it is not unusual to use a large coloured stimulus as an alternative to a smaller white stimulus. This is not, strictly speaking, colour perimetry. The same result could have just as easily been obtained with a desaturated white stimulus. This confusion has led some clinicians to discredit the value of colour perimetry by claiming that you can always detect a defect with white stimuli when one is present with a coloured stimulus.

Coloured stimuli and retinal pathologies

Because the response to coloured stimuli is dependent upon specific populations of receptors, any condition that selectively affects these populations will produce changes that are more readily apparent with coloured stimuli. For example, suppose we have a retinal condition that selectively damages the blue receptors. If we test the field with white stimuli then the response will be attenuated by an amount proportional to the contribution blue receptors make to the overall response of the retina, i.e. not much. If we now test with blue stimuli on a background of yellow light, which will attenuate the responses from both the green and blue receptors, then we will find a much greater sensitivity loss (see Chapter 4, p. 42 for more details of blue-on-yellow perimetry).

The next, and obvious, question to ask is are there any pathological conditions that selectively affect different populations of receptors? The answer is 'yes'; there are many conditions that affect one population more than another.

Retinitis pigmentosa selectively affects the rods before the cones. Coloured stimuli can be used to follow and differentiate between different forms of the disease (Massof and Finkelstein, 1981). Glaucoma selectively affects the blue cone mechanism and can produce more significant defects

when blue stimuli are used on a yellow background. Optic nerve disease has also been reported to produce more significant defects with coloured stimuli (Hart *et al.*, 1985).

Current use of coloured stimuli

Given that there is such strong evidence supporting the use of coloured stimuli the reader will perhaps be surprised to learn that it is not practised very frequently. Why? Well, one of the problems that perimetry faces is that there are just too many variables, a fact you may have already gathered having almost reached the end of this chapter, and there simply is not enough time to investigate them all. Standard techniques with white stimuli are already exceeding the limits of what patients can tolerate.

A second reason why colour perimetry is not more widely practised is the lack of suitable equipment. It is difficult to get equipment that is capable of presenting sufficiently intense coloured stimuli on coloured backgrounds. The papers cited above have largely been written by researchers who have either developed their own research perimeters or made major modifications to existing equipment.

A third reason is that while there is ample evidence to show that patients suspected of having glaucoma often have field defects that are selective to blue-on-yellow stimuli, the use of blue stimuli results in the test being particularly sensitive to changes in the crystalline lens. Further information on blue-on-yellow perimetry in glaucoma can be found in Chapter 4, p. 42.

PSYCHOLOGICAL FACTORS: THE FREQUENCY-OF-SEEING CURVE

Unfortunately, the sensitivity of the eye does not remain constant even after it has reached a steady state of adaptation. I say 'unfortunately' because if it did not vary then we would be able to get very accurate measures of the eye's peripheral sensitivity and be able to detect very small changes in sensitivity. As it is we can only be confident that the sensitivity has changed when the extent of change significantly exceeds variability.

One of the best ways of demonstrating how the eye's sensitivity changes with time is to plot what is known as a frequency-of-seeing curve. To do this, you find a range of intensities that straddle the patient's

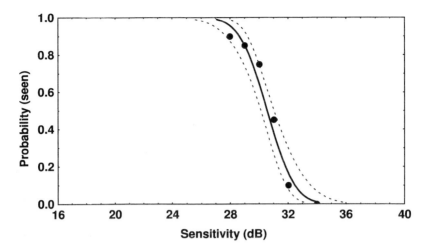

Fig. 2.13 *Frequency-of-seeing curve.*

sensitivity, i.e. the bright ones are above the patient's threshold and the dim ones are below it. You then choose half a dozen or so intensity levels between these two values and present stimuli over and over again, in a random manner, at all the chosen intensity levels. You then plot the percentage of times that the stimulus was seen at each of the intensity levels. At the high intensity levels the percentage seen will be close to 100 while at the dim levels it will be close to 0%. When you join all the values together, you should get an 'S' shaped curve like the one shown in Figure 2.13. This type of curve is known as an ogive.

There are several important points to make about the shape of this curve. The first is that its gradient is a measure of variability. The steeper it is, the less variability there is and the easier it is going to be to detect a small change in sensitivity. There are three important factors that affect the gradient of the frequency-of-seeing curve:[1]

(1) The patient. Some patients are simply more variable than others and there is not a lot that the perimetrist can do about it.

(2) The amount of perimetric experience. More experienced patients generally have steeper gradients. This is one reason why many of the psychophysical papers report data on very small highly trained groups of subjects.

[1] Variability in the results from a visual field test is also influenced by the examination strategy.

(3) The sensitivity of the eye. The gradient of the frequency-of-seeing curve reduces, variability increases, when the sensitivity is low. Figure 2.14 shows two frequency-of-seeing curves recorded during the same session on an eye with glaucomatous visual field loss. At one location, where the sensitivity is normal, the gradient of the frequency-of-seeing curve is steep while at the other, where the sensitivity is depressed, the gradient is shallow.

Gradient of frequency-of-seeing curve versus sensitivity

The data given in Figure 2.15 show the relationship between variability (gradient of the frequency-of-seeing curve) and sensitivity (Henson *et al.*, 2000a). It can be seen that as the sensitivity decreases (lower dB values) the variability increases. Plotted on this graph are data from patients with glaucomatous, ocular hypertensive and normal eyes. If we take patients with normal eyes, then we find that as you move into the peripheral field, where the sensitivity is lower, there is an increase in variability. In patients with glaucoma, when we examine a point where the sensitivity is normal the variability is similar to that of a normal eye and yet when we test a point where the sensitivity has been reduced by the pathology we find that the variability has been increased. The relationship between sensitivity and

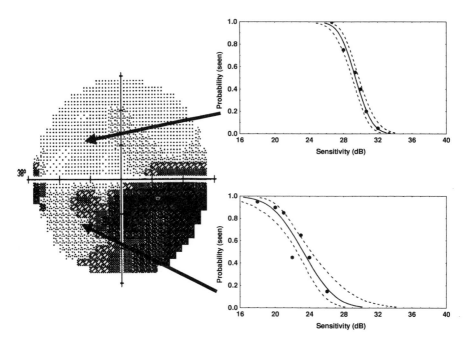

Fig. 2.14 *Two frequency-of-seeing curves: one from a part of the visual field where the sensitivity is normal and one from a region where the sensitivity is depressed.*

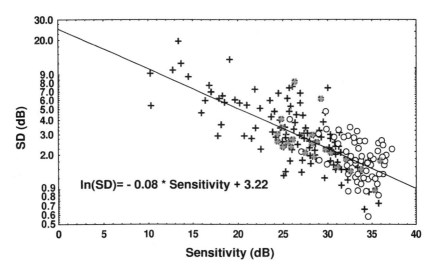

Fig. 2.15 *The relationship between variability (gradient of the frequency-of-seeing curve) and sensitivity. Each point represents a single test location in an eye which is normal (○), has glaucoma (+), or ocular hypertension (✳).*

variability is the same for normal and glaucomatous eyes. In fact, recent work on eyes with optic neuritis has shown that the same relationship exists for this pathology (Henson *et al.*, 2000b).

CONCLUDING REMARKS

Perimetry is concerned with establishing, at a whole series of retinal locations, whether a patient's differential light threshold is within the normal range of values.

This chapter has discussed how this measurement is sensitive to a large number of parameters, which often interact with each other in a highly complex manner.

While these interactions are of interest to the perimetrist, in that they may enable defects to be detected earlier, they at present provide the perimetrist with an 'embarras de richesses'. There are too many parameters and not enough time to investigate them all. There has, therefore, been a tendency amongst clinical perimetrists to try to rationalize things. More and more perimetrists are concentrating on using one or two strategies in which presentation time, stimulus size, background intensity and stimulus colour are all fixed, the only variables being stimulus intensity and retinal location. To these perimetrists the advantages of having a consistent form of perimetric examination outweigh the advantages of changing the parameters.

REFERENCES

Calkins J.L., Hochheimer B.F. and D'Anna S.A. (1980) Potential hazards from specific ophthalmic devices. *Vis Res*, 20, 1039–1053.

Dubois-Poulson A. and Magis C. (1959) La dysharmonie photometrique dans le champ visuel des glaucomateux. *Doc Ophthalmol*, 13, 186–302.

Flanagan J.G., Trope G.E., Popick W. and Grover A. (1991) Perimetric isolation of the SWS cones in OHT and early POAG. In *Perimetry Update 1990/91* (eds Mills R.P. and Heijl A.). Kugler & Ghedini, Amsterdam, pp. 331–337.

Glezer V.D. (1965) The receptive fields of the retina. *Vis Res*, 5, 479–525.

Goldmann H. (1945) Cited in Tate G.W. and Lynn J.R. (1977) *Principles of Quantitative Perimetry*. Grune & Stratton, New York.

Greve E.L. (1973) *Single and Multiple Stimulus Static Perimetry in Glaucoma; the Two Phases of Visual Field Examination*. Dr W Junk, The Hague.

Guilford J.P. (1954) *Psychometric Methods*. Tata McGraw Hill, New Delhi.

Hallett P.E. (1963) Spatial summation. *Vis Res*, 3, 9–24.

Hart W.M., Gordon M.O., Silverman S.E. and Kass M.A. (1991) Equiluminant blue/yellow color contrast perimetry (CCP) in high risk ocular hypertension (OHT) and glaucoma (POAG). In *Perimetry Update 1990/91* (eds Mills R.P. and Heijl A.). Kugler & Ghedini, Amsterdam, pp. 325–329.

Hart W.M., Kosmorsky G. and Burde R.M. (1995) Color perimetry of central scotomas in diseases of the macular and optic nerve. *Doc Ophthalmol Proc Series*, 42, 239–245.

Henson D.B. and Anderson R. (1989) Thresholds using single and multiple stimulus presentations. In *Perimetry Update 1988/89* (ed. Heijl A.). Kugler & Ghedini, Amsterdam, pp. 191–196.

Henson D. B., Chaudry S. and Artes P. H. (2000a) The relationship between sensitivity and variability in normal and glaucomatous visual fields. In *Perimetry Update 1998/1999* (eds Wall M. and Wild S. M.). Kugler and Ghedini, Amsterdam, pp. 95–101.

Henson D. B., Chaudry S., Artes P. H., Faragher E. B. and Ansons A. (2000b) Response variability in the visual field: Comparison of optic neuritis, glaucoma, ocular hypertension and normal eyes. *Invest Ophthalmol Vis Sci*, 41, 417–421.

Johnson C.A., Adams A.J. and Lewis R.A. (1989) Automated perimetry of short-wavelength mechanisms in glaucoma and ocular hypertension. In *Perimetry Update 1988/89* (ed Heijl A.). Kugler & Ghedini, Amsterdam, pp. 31–38.

Lie I. (1980) Visual detection and resolution as a function of retinal locus. *Vis Res*, 20, 967–974.

Massof R.W. and Finkelstein D. (1981) Subclassification of retinitis pigmentosa from two-color scotopic static perimetry. *Doc Ophthalmol Proc Series*, 26, 219–225.

Rouf J.A.J. (1966) On the relationship between the threshold of short flashes, the flicker–fusion frequency and visual latency. Institute for Perception Research, Eindhoven, The Netherlands, Annual report number 1, pp. 69–77.

Rouf J.A.J. and Meulenbrugge N.J. (1967) The quantitative relationship between flash threshold and the flicker–fusion boundary for centrally fixated fields. Institute for Perceptual Research, Eindhoven, The Netherlands, Annual report number 2, pp. 133–139.

Sloan L.L. (1961) Area and luminance of test object as variables in examination of the visual field by projection perimetry. *Vis Res*, 1, 121–138.

Wilson M.E. (1970) Invariant features of spatial summation with changing locus in the visual field. *J Physiol*, 207, 611–622.

3 Strategies used in examining the visual field

INTRODUCTION

To the newcomer, one of the most confusing aspects of visual field investigation must surely be the overwhelming number of different ways in which the visual field can be examined. Is it really necessary to have all these different strategies for investigating the visual field? Cannot the perimetric community decide which strategy is the best and then do away with the rest?

The short answer to these questions is 'no'. Different visual field strategies are necessary because the objectives of a visual field examination vary from one situation to another. What might be an ideal strategy for one situation could be totally inappropriate for another. For example, a neurologist examining a patient with a suspected pituitary tumour has a very different need to that of an optometrist who wishes to quickly check that his patient does not have any significant visual field loss. Different examination strategies have been devised to meet these very different objectives.

While different objectives clearly justify the need for several different examination strategies, it is now clear that some strategies have long outlived their usefulness. The one-level suprathreshold strategy is an obvious example. It has no advantage over an eccentrically compensated (gradient-adapted) suprathreshold strategy and has the major disadvantage of being either less sensitive or less specific. There is, therefore, some scope for the number of examination strategies to be reduced.

Before readers gets too excited about a future in which the number of examination strategies has been rationalised, they should bear in mind that the capacity of researchers to devise new strategies (which

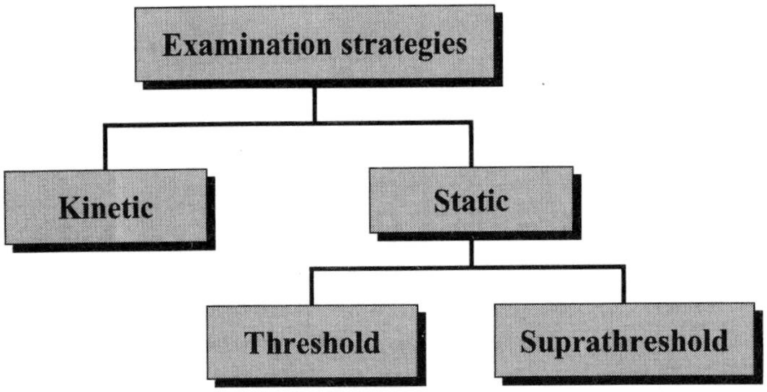

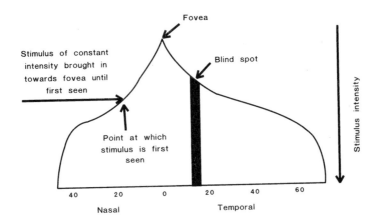

Fig. 3.1 *Classification of examination strategies.*

Fig. 3.2 *Profile of the visual field.*

invariably have some advantage or other for one group of perimetrists) is almost infinite. At the present time new examination strategies are being developed much faster than the old ones are being discarded. Newcomers to visual fields have, therefore, little option but to try to fathom out the relative merits of the various examination strategies before coming to a decision about which is the most appropriate for their particular situation. Before readers get too despondent, I should like to point out that the practice of perimetry is invariably quite straightforward once that decision has been made.

This chapter covers all the major examination strategies that use classic white spot stimuli. It does not cover confrontation tests, Amsler grids, frequency-doubling perimetry and blue–yellow perimetry. Details of these alternative test strategies, along with others, can be found in Chapter 4. This chapter will

also not include details on how to conduct a visual field examination. This information will be found in Chapter 10.

Classic white spot examination strategies can be divided into two main categories (see Figure 3.1):

1. kinetic strategies, in which a stimulus of constant size and intensity is moved around the visual field (the stimulus moves, hence the term kinetic);
2. and static strategies in which the stimulus remains stationary (hence the term static).

KINETIC EXAMINATION STRATEGIES

Kinetic examination strategies rely upon the fact that the centre of the visual field is normally more sensitive than the periphery (see Figure 3.2). A stimulus that is a little too weak to be seen at the edge of the visual field

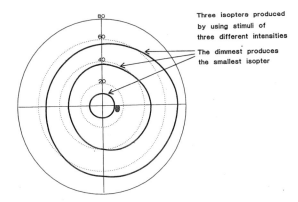

Three isopters produced by using stimuli of three different intensities

The dimmest produces the smallest isopter

Fig. 3.3 *Three isopters produced by the kinetic strategy.*

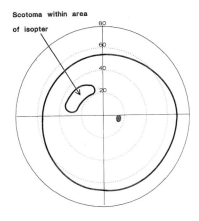

Scotoma within area of isopter

Fig. 3.4 *Isopter diagram showing an upper nasal scotoma.*

becomes visible as it is brought towards the centre. With the kinetic examination strategies the perimetrist selects a stimulus of a given size and intensity and moves it from outside the visual field towards its centre, noting the position at which it first becomes visible. This is repeated along a series of different meridians and the points at which the stimulus first became visible are then joined together by a line which is called an isopter (see Figure 3.3). Scotoma (see Figure 3.4) within the area of an isopter are detected by continuing to move the stimulus towards the centre of the visual field after it has first been detected. The patient is asked to report if, at any time, it disappears.

The perimetrist can repeat the whole process with stimuli of differing size and/or intensity, in order to build up a map of the patient's visual field, such as that given in Figure 3.3. Note how in this figure the isopters look like contour lines on a relief map. This

analogy between isopter diagrams and relief maps is frequently brought out in the terminology used by perimetrists. It is common for perimetrists to talk about the 'island of vision', the 'height' of the sensitivity profile and the 'depth' of a defect.

Kinetic perimetry is normally conducted with a bowl perimeter or tangent screen, typical ones being the Goldmann bowl perimeter and the Bjerrum tangent screen. The major difference between these two classes of instrument is that tangent screens only examine the central 25–30 degrees of the visual field, while bowl perimeters are capable of measuring out to an eccentricity of up to 90 degrees. As tangent screens are normally placed further away from the patient than the surface of bowl perimeters – 1 m versus 30 cm for most instruments – there is a greater magnification of the central field that can lead to more accurate plotting of central defects.

Kinetic examination strategies were very popular in the early days of perimetry. They have, however, been largely replaced by static techniques over the past 10 years. Why should this be so? What are the disadvantages of kinetic strategies and for that matter what are their advantages?

Advantages of kinetic examination strategies

One of the major advantages of kinetic examination strategies is that the perimetrist has almost total control over the examination. The perimetrist can examine as much or as little as he or she wishes. The field can be examined in whatever order the perimetrist wishes, with particular attention being paid to specific regions of the field or whole regions being completely ignored. Finally, the perimetrist can move the stimulus in whatever direction, and at whatever speed, he or she likes.

This flexibility allows perimetrists to adjust their examination technique to the specific problems presented by each patient. The perimetrist can slow down the examination when the patient appears flustered, or the patient who begins to make errors. The perimetrist can also reduce any variability in the results by repeating measurements that appear unusual.

This degree of flexibility can be extremely valuable. When re-examining a patient who has an established defect the previous field chart can be used as a template to quickly check whether the extent of field loss has changed. I am not suggesting that this should be done in all cases where a patient is being re-examined, for clearly there is a need to establish whether any new defects have occurred. I present this simply as an example of how flexible kinetic strategies can be.

Disadvantages of kinetic examination strategies

The major disadvantage of kinetic examination strategies is that they are relatively time consuming and do not lend themselves well to a quick screening of the visual field.

A second disadvantage is that they appear to be less sensitive when it comes to the detection of scotoma (Drance, 1969; Greve and Verduin, 1977). It has been suggested (somewhat facetiously) that if one didn't know where the blind spot was one would be unlikely to find it in a routine kinetic examination. One explanation for this lowered sensitivity is that when moving a stimulus within the boundary of an isopter the perimetrist is relying upon the patient to report if it disappears or dims. The majority of patients want to be helpful and want to be able to see the stimulus. As a consequence of this they often fail to report or notice the momentary disappearance that occurs when the stimulus passes through a scotoma. Lapses of attention by the patient, which are not uncommon during the fairly tedious procedure of a visual field examination, may also result in the patient failing to recognize that the stimulus has disappeared. The ideal examination strategy would be one where any lapses of attention resulted in the assumption that a defect exists rather than, as in the case of kinetic perimetry, that the field is normal.

The flexibility of kinetic examination strategies, which was cited as one of its advantages, can, ironically, also be seen as a disadvantage. When several different perimetrists are employed to collect visual field data, there is a danger that they will not examine the visual field in exactly the same way. In these situations, it can be difficult to decide whether changes in the visual field are the product of changes in the technique of examination or real changes in the patient's visual field.

Role of kinetic strategies

So, what is the current role of the kinetic strategy?

Flexibility remains one of its greatest strengths. Kinetic examination strategies are, therefore, ideal in an environment where a great deal of flexibility is of value, e.g. in a neurological clinic where one minute you are looking for a hemianopia, the next a central loss and the next an enlarged blind spot. If, on the other hand, perimetry is going to be practised in an environment where a large number of patients have similar defects and the ideal form of examination can be more precisely defined, e.g. a glaucoma clinic, then this flexibility becomes redundant and could even be considered a disadvantage.

Kinetic perimetry is also used to map the residual field of patients who are known to have severe visual field loss. An example would be a patient who has only a small central island of vision that does not extend beyond the central 5 degrees. In such a situation the use of static examination strategies would result in many undetected stimuli and because the stimuli are often placed on a relatively coarse matrix would not accurately map the residual field. Kinetic techniques would give greater precision without unnecessary frustration.

The kinetic strategy is also found to be useful in patients who, for a variety of reasons, cannot cope with static techniques. This would include young children and those with attention problems.

If the perimetrist is intending to screen a large number of patients, either as part of a routine ophthalmological examination, or in a mass screening programme, then the time taken to perform a kinetic examination is a big disincentive.

STATIC EXAMINATION STRATEGIES

Under the general heading of static examination strategies falls a large number of different field testing techniques. While some may have been developed to quickly screen the visual field, others have been developed to give detailed information concerning the depth and extent of any visual field loss. They are lumped together under the term 'static' simply because the stimuli in these strategies do not move.

Static examination strategies have over the past few years become increasingly popular and in many clinics have almost entirely replaced kinetic ones. This change has resulted from a variety of factors, among which are the following:

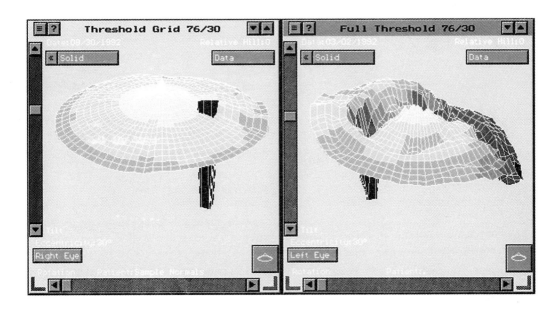

Fig. 3.5 *A surface plot of threshold data as an example of how computers can present visual field data in novel ways. Result from Field View.*

(1) Operator independence. Static examination strategies are, on the whole, less sensitive to operator variability. Some are almost entirely independent of the operator, whose task is simply to explain the test, align the patient and start the program.

(2) Speed. Static strategies can be used to rapidly screen the visual field.

(3) Numerical analysis. The results from static measures of the threshold lend themselves particularly well to a wide variety of analytical techniques. These techniques are used to reduce the relatively large amount of numerical data obtained from a static examination to one or more numbers that summarize the extent of the defect. They can also be used to analyse any differences that have occurred between visits and establish whether or not these are significant.

(4) Computer control. Computers are very good at performing routine repetitive tasks, such as the presentation and collection of visual field data. They never, unlike us mere mortals, get bored. The advent of low cost computers which can collect, store and graphically present the results from static investigations has given the static

examination strategies a tremendous boost. In addition to this, computers can display the results of an examination in novel ways that can make the interpretation of results easier (see Figure 3.5).

Two very important parameters within a static test are the number and the position of stimuli. Obviously, these two parameters have a major role to play in both test sensitivity and test duration. This relationship will be covered in detail in Chapter 8.

Static examination strategies can also differ in the actual nature of the test. Some static strategies derive an estimate of the eye's threshold at a whole series of different test locations. These are known as threshold tests. Others present their stimuli at an intensity that is calculated to be slightly above the patient's threshold and simply record whether or not the stimuli are seen. These are known as suprathreshold tests (see Figure 3.1)

Each static strategy has its own particular advantages and disadvantages. Some, such as the suprathreshold strategies, are ideally suited for rapid screening while others, such as the threshold tests, are widely used for monitoring the visual field.

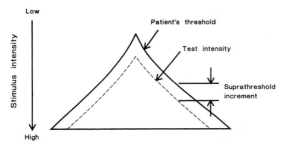

Fig. 3.6 *Profile of visual field showing the suprathreshold increment.*

Suprathreshold strategies

In a suprathreshold examination strategy the stimuli are initially presented at an intensity which is calculated to be above the patient's threshold (see Figure 3.6). If the stimuli are seen then it is assumed that no significant defect exists. This strategy has largely been developed as a screening procedure for conditions such as glaucoma. In comparison to other examination strategies, e.g. threshold strategies, they can test a far greater number of locations in the same amount of time or, if you like, the same number of locations in far less time. This is simply a reflection of the fact that most locations[1] are only tested once.

The suprathreshold examination strategy is ideally suited to computerization and automation. A computer can be programmed to present stimuli in a predetermined order and to record the patient's responses through some form of response button. At the end of the test it can produce a printout showing the positions at which stimuli were missed. The clinician can then decide whether to conduct any further examination.

There are many different types of suprathreshold strategies. To try to help the student understand the relationship between these, Figure 3.7 has attempted to bring most of them together in a single diagram. Each level of this diagram represents an option for the perimetrist. Do I want to do a 'one-level' or an 'eccentrically compensated' test? Do I want to do a 'single stimulus' or 'multiple stimulus' test etc? The advantages and disadvantages (costs and benefits) of each of these decisions will be dealt with in the following sections of this chapter. A definition for each of the terms used will be found in the Glossary.

[1] Locations are normally tested a second time if they are missed on the first occasion. The number of repeat presentations will be dependent upon the extent of any visual field loss.

One word of warning. This diagram is not complete and never can be. For no sooner does a text like this go to print than someone brings out a new form of suprathreshold test. A second word of warning. The names given to all the different static tests do vary from one text to another and from one instrument manual to another. So be warned: an 'eccentrically compensated' test may be called a 'gradient adapted' test in your field perimeter's manual!

Selection of the test intensity

Selection of the test intensity is an important part of a suprathreshold test. If the intensity is set too high then there is a danger that shallow defects will be missed. The test becomes insensitive to shallow defects, and produces too many false negatives. On the other hand, if the test intensity is set too low, close to the threshold of the patient, then a large number of patients with normal visual fields will miss stimuli (see Figure 3.8). In this case, the test has a low specificity and produces too many false positives. The simple rule describing the effects of altering the suprathreshold increment is:

(1) The higher the suprathreshold increment the higher the specificity and the lower the sensitivity.

(2) The lower the suprathreshold increment the lower the specificity and the higher the sensitivity.

Chauhan (1987) used a mathematical technique called information theory to look at the effects of varying the test intensity with respect to the patient's threshold. He found that information peaked when the test intensity was 6 dB above the patient's threshold and concluded that the ideal suprathreshold increment was 6 dB. The majority of instruments currently being used recommend that you test at intensities calculated to be between 4 and 6 dB above the patient's threshold.

Eccentrically compensated or one-level suprathreshold tests?

At the adaptation levels used in perimetry (lower photopic), the foveal region of the visual field is more sensitive than the periphery (see Chapter 2, *Background luminance and the sensitivity profile*, p. 10 for more details). To retain a constant relationship between the intensity of the stimuli and the threshold, it is necessary for the stimulus intensity to

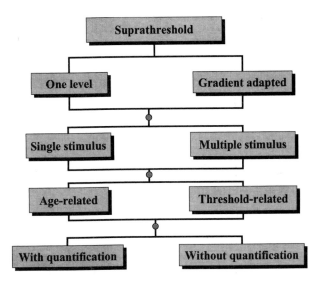

Fig. 3.7 *Classification of static suprathreshold strategies.*

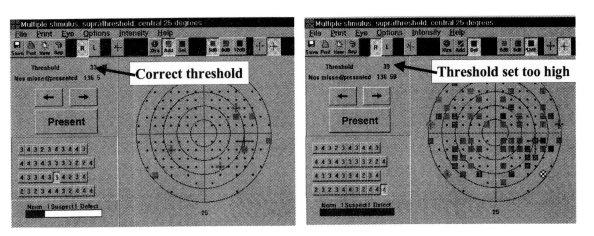

Fig. 3.8 *The effect of setting the threshold too high. Result from Henson Pro perimeter.*

vary with test location. Such strategies are known as 'eccentrically compensated' or 'gradient-adapted'. A strategy that does not take into account this change in sensitivity with eccentricity, i.e. one that presents all the stimuli at the same intensity irrespective of their eccentricity, is known as a 'one-level' test. Figure 3.9 diagrammatically represents how test results can be affected by the use of an eccentrically compensated strategy as opposed to a one-level one. Depending upon the selected suprathreshold increment, one-level tests will either be less sensitive (more false negatives) or less specific (more false positives) than eccentrically compensated tests.

The majority of instruments that incorporate eccentrically compensated suprathreshold strategies use a database of normal values to calculate the test intensity.

Single or multiple stimulus suprathreshold tests?

In a single stimulus suprathreshold strategy stimuli are presented one at a time and patients are asked to press a response button each time they see a stimulus. The test is fully automated in that once started there is no need for the perimetrist to do anything other than give the odd encouraging comment to the patient and to make sure that things are progressing smoothly. Single

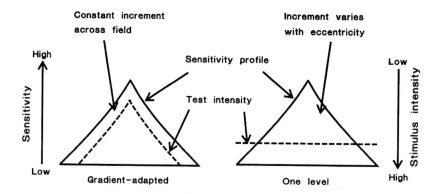

Fig. 3.9   *The difference between one level and eccentrically compensated strategies.*

stimulus tests incorporate false positive catch trials (see *Variability*, p. 37) to break up the long sequences of positive responses. Without these catch trials there is the danger that patients will simply get into a rhythm of pressing the button after each presentation, even when they do not see a stimulus.

Several instruments, such as the Dicon LD400 and the Henson range of instruments (details on these instruments can be found in Chapter 11) are also capable of presenting patterns of 2, 3 or 4 stimuli at a time, the patient's task being to verbally report to the perimetrist the number of seen stimuli. If the number reported is correct the perimetrist goes straight onto the next pattern. The number of stimuli varies from pattern to pattern in a manner that the patient cannot predict. If the number reported is incorrect then the perimetrist asks the patient to report at what locations the stimuli were seen. It is then the perimetrist's task to establish the location/s of any missed stimuli and to either mark them on the chart or enter them into the computer. This type of test is often called semi-automated because while many of the operations are automated (selection of test location, number of stimuli etc.) the perimetrist is still responsible for asking the questions and keying in the responses.

One of the major advantages of multiple stimulus strategies is that they are faster than single stimulus ones, taking approximately half the amount of time for the same number of stimuli.

Another advantage is that they promote a dialogue between the patient and the perimetrist. This has certain psychological advantages (De Jong *et al.*, 1985) and has been shown to produce threshold estimates which have a smaller standard deviation,

i.e. are subject to less variability, than single stimulus strategies (Henson and Anderson, 1989).

A disadvantage of the multiple stimulus strategy arises when a patient has a large area of defect affecting many of the stimuli. In these situations the perimetrist has to ask the patient to identify the stimulus locations in a high proportion of the patterns. This process slows down the test and can lead to a certain amount of frustration and anxiety in the patient who is continually being reminded of all the stimuli he or she cannot see.

In summary, multiple stimulus techniques are ideal in a screening environment where the majority of patients have normal visual fields. In this situation, the advantages experienced by the majority of patients outweigh the disadvantages experienced by the few.

Age-related, or threshold-related, suprathreshold tests?

At the onset of this section a suprathreshold strategy was defined as one in which stimuli are presented at an intensity calculated to be above the patient's threshold. But how do we know what the patient's threshold is in order to calculate the suprathreshold test intensity? The short answer is that we don't. We either have to assume a value or estimate it from a series of measurements.

There are currently two techniques that are widely used for estimating the patient's threshold.

(1) The first is to base the threshold estimate on the patient's age. This strategy is known as an 'age-related suprathreshold test'. It is well

known that the sensitivity of the eye decreases with age, declining at a rate of approximately 0.6 dB/decade (see Chapter 5). It is, therefore, fairly simple for a set of tables to be attached to or incorporated into the instrument which can be used to calculate the best test intensity on the basis of the patient's age. The advantages of this technique are its simplicity and speed. A disadvantage is that within any particular age group not all patients will have the same sensitivity. This is particularly so in the older age groups where factors such as cataracts can have an effect upon the patient's threshold. It should be recalled that it is the older age groups that most frequently develop visual field loss and are, therefore, most frequently subjected to visual field examination.

(2) The second option is to precede the suprathreshold examination with a short routine that estimates the patient's threshold. This strategy is known as a 'threshold-related suprathreshold strategy'. It is currently the most popular suprathreshold strategy and compensates for any variations in sensitivity within a particular age group. Clearly, there are many different ways in which the initial threshold estimate can be established and, at present, there does not seem to be any consensus as to which is the most appropriate. It is a little ironic that while the majority of perimetrists have agreed that a threshold-related strategy is the best one to use they have not agreed on the best way to derive the threshold estimate. A recommended technique for establishing the threshold can be found in Chapter 10.

Time is an important parameter when deciding which of these two options to choose. The threshold-related strategy takes longer to perform than the age-related one. The price of a more accurate threshold estimate is, therefore, an increase in test time. The designers of suprathreshold strategies, therefore, have to carefully weigh several factors:

(a) the extent of the suprathreshold increment, which controls the sensitivity and the specificity of the test;

(b) the accuracy of the initial threshold estimate;

(c) and the time taken to make the initial threshold estimate.

Two studies have looked at the accuracy of different techniques of establishing the suprathreshold test intensity. In the first study (Henson and Anderson, 1991) age-related measures were found to differ from accurate threshold measures with a standard deviation of 1.7 dB (this means that over 30% of estimates would be in error by ≥ 1.7 dB and 5% by ≥ 3.4 dB). Given that the suprathreshold increment is normally between 4 and 6 dB, relying on an age setting is likely to lead to a significant number of false positive test results. A simple multiple stimulus staircase technique (stepping the intensity down in 1 dB steps until the patient cannot see any of the stimuli) was found to give much more accurate threshold estimates (SD 0.8 dB).

The second study (Henson *et al.*, 1999) looked at the single stimulus threshold related technique that is currently incorporated in the Humphrey Visual Field Analyzer. This technique uses a full-threshold technique at four locations in the visual field and then takes the second most sensitive result as a basis for calculating the suprathreshold test intensity. An upper limit is placed on the intensity to guard against it being set too high. Henson *et al.* found that the SD of the threshold estimate was anywhere between 1.4 and 1.9 dB (depending upon whether or not there was a visual field defect). This result is only marginally better than the age-related technique; in fact it is worse in eyes with some pre-existing damage. They concluded that there was a need to develop better techniques for establishing the threshold at the onset of single stimulus suprathreshold tests and that until that time practitioners should be wary of results in which the threshold-related value differs significantly from the expected normal for the patient's age. It is important to emphasize that this problem is unique to single stimulus fully automated tests. The algorithms used in the semi-automated multiple stimulus techniques currently give a more precise estimate of the threshold and hence do not suffer from this problem.

Suprathreshold tests with or without quantification
Suprathreshold strategies also vary on the basis of what happens when a stimulus is missed (see Figure 3.10).

(1) A suprathreshold test without quantification. This is the most basic form of suprathreshold test: stimuli are either seen or missed and

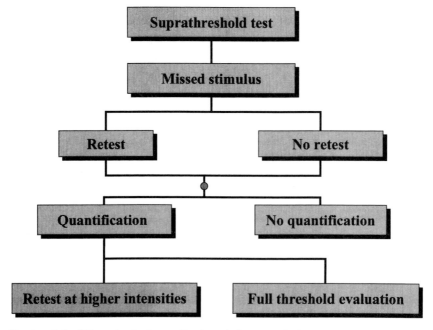

Fig. 3.10 *Classification of the different levels of quantification which are available with suprathreshold test strategies.*

marked accordingly on the printout. This is a suprathreshold test without quantification.

(2) A suprathreshold test with repeats. A slightly more sophisticated form will automatically retest any missed stimuli at the same intensity. If it is seen on the second presentation, then it is assumed that the initial miss was a false positive. (It should be remembered that in a non-selected population, a missed stimulus is more likely to be a false positive than a true positive.) The output of this type of test is essentially the same as the former except each marked miss has been missed on two occasions rather than one. It is generally accepted that a test with repeats is significantly better and well worth the extra examination time.

(3) A suprathreshold test with quantification. An even more sophisticated type of suprathreshold test will present missed stimuli at higher intensities to obtain some measure of defect depth. There are two widely used versions:

(a) those that retest defect areas at higher suprathreshold increments – in these instances defects are normally graded into three or four categories and the field charts marked accordingly;

(b) those that retest defect areas with a threshold strategy in order to get an estimate of defect depth at damaged test locations.

The value of different levels of quantification is subject to a certain amount of disagreement. Some would argue that once suspicion has been aroused from the results of a suprathreshold test, the patient should be subjected to a threshold examination. Others would argue that you can reliably quantify the extent of visual field loss with suprathreshold examination strategies and that threshold tests, of equivalent duration, give very little additional information.

At present there is no conclusive evidence one way or the other as to the relative value of these two types of examination strategy. Those comparisons that have been published tend not to compare like with like, e.g. they compare the accuracy of a 5 minute suprathreshold screening test with a 15 minute threshold test.

Threshold strategies

There is, understandably, some confusion concerning what a threshold strategy is. Pragmatically, a threshold strategy is one in which the threshold is estimated at a series of different test locations. The confusion arises because there are many different ways of deriving a threshold estimate (for a review of these see Guilford, 1984) and, therefore, many different types of threshold test. Confusion is further fostered by the use of loose terminology. The term full-threshold test is normally interpreted as a particular bracketing strategy (see below), however, it is occasionally inappropriately used to describe other threshold strategies.

The results obtained from any threshold technique will be prone to a certain amount of error, i.e. difference between the true threshold at any given location and the measured threshold. The smaller this error is, the better the technique. Generally speaking, the more elaborate, and hence time consuming, a technique is the more accurate is its threshold estimate. The problem for perimetry (and indeed for many other clinical measures) is that time is not unlimited. Patients cannot be expected (even if the other facilities exist) to spend long periods of time undergoing the demanding task of a visual field investigation. If a limit is set on examination time, then the longer it takes to derive a threshold measure at each test location the fewer locations can be tested. One of the prime objectives in designing a threshold strategy is, therefore, to optimize for both time and accuracy.

The five most widely used threshold strategies are the full-threshold strategy, the fast-threshold strategy, the dynamic strategy, Tendency Orientated Perimetry (TOP) and the recently developed Swedish Interactive Thresholding Algorithm (SITA). All five strategies share the following characteristics:

1. Randomization of stimulus test location. Threshold tests require several measurements to be made at each test location. These do not occur one after another but are mixed up with the presentations at the other test locations. This mixing up makes it impossible for the patient to predict the location of the next stimulus and thus discourages fixation errors.
2. Incorporate estimates of fixation losses (by catch trails), false positive errors and false negative errors. These are described in more detail in *Variability*, p. 37.

The full-threshold strategy

The full-threshold strategy was first described by Spahr (1975) and Bebie *et al.* (1976b) and incorporated

in the first computerized perimeter, the Octopus 201. It has since been adopted by almost all computerized static perimeters.

The developers theoretically evaluated a number of different psychophysical strategies and concluded that the optimal one (time and precision) was a 'two reversal staircase' in which the step size reduced from 4 dB to 2 dB after the first reversal.

The best way to understand this strategy is by working through a number of examples. In Figure 3.11 there are four examples of how this examination strategy would establish the threshold at a test location. The initial intensity at which the target is presented is based either upon the age of the patient or, if available, the threshold of neighbouring test locations.

Example 1. In this example, the first presentation is not seen. The intensity of the second presentation is therefore 4 dB above that of the first. The second presentation is again not seen and the third is therefore presented at a further 4 dB above that of the second. The third presentation is seen, this marks the first reversal of the patient's responses, and the fourth presentation is, therefore, presented at 2 dB below that of the third. This fourth presentation is not seen and the fifth presentation is therefore presented at 2 dB above the fourth. This presentation is seen, which marks the second reversal. The threshold is taken as lying between the fourth and fifth presentations.

Example 2. The first presentation is seen and the second is therefore presented at 4 dB below that of the first. The second presentation is not seen (the first reversal) and the third presentation is presented at 2 dB above that of the second. The third presentation is seen, the second reversal, and the threshold is, therefore, taking as lying between the second and third presentations.

Example 3. The first presentation is not seen and the second is therefore presented at 4 dB above that of the first. The second presentation is seen (first reversal) and the third presentation is 2 dB below that of the second. The third presentation is seen, therefore, the fourth is presented at 2 dB below that of the third. The fourth presentation is not seen (second reversal) and the threshold is taken as lying between the third and fourth presentations.

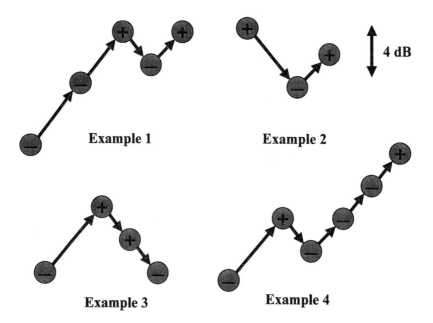

Fig. 3.11   *Examples of how the threshold is established in the full threshold strategy. Plus indicates that the stimulus was seen, minus that it was missed.*

Example 4. The first presentation is not seen and the second presentation is 4 dB above that of the first. The second presentation is seen (first reversal) and the third presentation is, therefore, presented at 2 dB below that of the second. The third presentation is not seen and the fourth is presented at 2 dB above that of the third. The fourth presentation is not seen and the fifth is presented at 2 dB above that of the fourth. The fifth presentation is not seen and the sixth is therefore presented at 2 dB above that of the fifth. The sixth presentation is seen (second reversal) and the threshold is taken as lying between the fifth and sixth presentations. In this example, the patient's response to the second presentation appears to have been a false positive which has been corrected by the following 2 dB steps. False positives or false negatives occurring after the first reversal will result in errors in the threshold estimate.

The full-threshold strategy of the Humphrey Visual Field Analyzer differs from that for the Octopus in that rather than set the threshold as lying between the intensities of the last seen and last missed responses it sets it to the intensity of the last seen response.

The full-threshold strategy has become a standard technique for monitoring glaucoma patients and as

such has been used in a large number of research projects. It is not, however, ideal. It suffers from four major drawbacks:

1. Long test time. Actual test times (the time the patient spends responding to stimuli) is normally given as a little over 13 minutes per eye (Wild *et al.*, 1999). Total test time (including setting the patient up, giving instruction, demonstrating the program and the occasional break) is closer to 20 min/eye.

2. Demanding task. This strategy is very demanding for the patient. They are continuously being asked whether or not they can see a stimulus that is very close to their threshold and, by definition, is going to be difficult to see. Patients find this task difficult and exhausting.

3. Poor repeatability. Threshold estimates, especially at locations where there is some loss in sensitivity, show large amounts of variability. This makes it very difficult to differentiate between progressive loss and random noise (see Chapter 3, *The SITA Strategies*, p. 36 and Chapter 2, *Psychological factors: the frequency-of-seeing curve*, p. 19).

4. There is a significant learning effect. Results

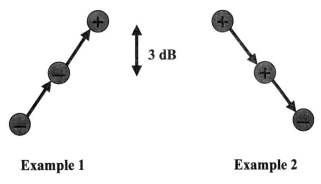

Example 1   **Example 2**

Fig. 3.12 *Examples of how the threshold is established in the fast threshold strategy. Plus indicates that the stimulus was seen, minus that it was missed.*

from the second examination often differ from the first as the patient gets to know what is required of them. It is recommended that the results from the first examination be disregarded for the purposes of detecting progressive changes in the visual field.

The fast-threshold strategy
This strategy was designed to overcome the first drawback mentioned above (long test time). Rather than use a two-reversal staircase it uses just one reversal and rather than have two step sizes (4 and 2 dB) it uses a single step size of 3 dB. This strategy is much simpler than the full-threshold strategy. Stimuli which are not seen are gradually increased (3 dB steps) until seen and those initially seen are gradually decreased in intensity until not seen (see Figure 3.12).

While this strategy achieves its objective of being faster than the full-threshold strategy (it saves approx. 5.5 min/eye) it does so at the cost of reduced accuracy (Glass *et al.*, 1995). Repeat measures of the threshold with this strategy show an increase in variability of between 20 and 43% over that of the full-threshold strategy (value dependent upon the patient response characteristics, see Chapter 2, *Psychological factors: the frequency-of-seeing curve*, p. 19).

The fast-threshold strategy is often used in situations where patients find it difficult to complete the full-threshold test. It is also used when resources make it difficult to routinely use full-threshold perimetry and yet there is still a need for a threshold test result.

The dynamic strategy
The dynamic strategy was developed by Weber following his research on the relationship between variability and sensitivity (Weber and Rau, 1992). Weber established that the variability of a patient's responses increased as the sensitivity of the tested location reduced (see Chapter 2, *Gradient of frequency-of-seeing curve versus sensitivity*, p. 20).

This has important implications for the calculation of the optimal (speed and accuracy) thresholding algorithm. In the original work of Bebie and Spahr (Bebie *et al.* 1976b), which led to the development of the full-threshold strategy, variability was set to match that found at a test location of normal sensitivity. If you increase the amount of variability and repeat Bebie and Spahr's calculations, the ideal step size increases.

The logical conclusion is that step sizes should increase as the estimated sensitivity reduces in order for the strategy to remain 'optimal'. This is exactly what the dynamic strategy does. The step size increases from 2 to 10 dB. Because the dynamic strategy remains optimal the number of presentations at locations where the sensitivity estimate is low is reduced, i.e. it reduces overall test time in comparison to the standard full-threshold strategy.

In theory the dynamic principle of varying step sizes could be combined with any number of reversals. In the current generation of Octopus perimeters a one-reversal staircase is used. By using a one-reversal option Octopus have further reduced the examination times (approx. 40% of the full-threshold strategy). One reversal techniques are, however, less accurate and hence the overall precision of the dynamic strategy is reduced. The Octopus programs allow retesting of all locations to improve repeatability (see Chapter 11, *Octopus Perimeters*, p. 151).

Tendency orientated perimetry (TOP)

Tendency orientated perimetry (TOP) was developed by González de la Rosa (González de la Rosa *et al.*, 1997) and is also incorporated in the Octopus range of perimeters (1-2-3 and 101).

TOP, rather than independently establishing the threshold at each test location combines the information from several locations, thereby reducing the overall test time. Each test location is in fact only tested once. The version incorporated within the current Octopus range of instruments uses the standard 30-2 pattern of stimuli (6 degree square matrix de-centred 3 degrees from the vertical and horizontal meridians, covering the central 30 degrees of the visual field). The 76 test locations are divided into 19 groups of 4.

The algorithm starts off by assuming the patient has a normal sensitivity at all test locations. One location in each group is then tested at an intensity equal to 50% of the normal age-matched value. The results from these 19 locations are used to recalculate the threshold estimates for all 76 test locations. This is repeated for the second, third and fourth locations in each group to derive the final threshold estimates. The size of the adjustments reduces after each round, being one-quarter of the normal threshold after the first round, reducing to one-sixteenth after the last.

At the end of the test, global indices, such as mean defect, are calculated. A clinical evaluation of this strategy (González de la Rosa *et al.*, 1997) has shown good correlations for global indices (>0.9) and for individual test locations (0.84). The excellent relationship between global indices owes much to the infrequent occurrence of small scotoma in glaucoma populations and brings into question whether coarser spatial test matrices might be just as sensitive as the standard 6 degree one (30-2 pattern). Visual field defects with tendency orientated perimetry have rounder edges and are shallower, giving a smoothed effect to the visual field.

The SITA strategies

The SITA (Swedish Interactive Thresholding Algorithm) is one of the latest developments in automated perimetry. It is only available on the Humphrey 700 series of instruments. The aim of its developers (Bengtsson *et al.*, 1997; Bengtsson and Heijl, 1998) was to create a faster thresholding algorithm whose repeatability was the same as that of the full-threshold strategy.

They have achieved this by writing a strategy which:

1. takes more account of prior knowledge;
2. does away with the need for false positive catch trials;
3. speeds up the rate of stimulus presentation in patients who respond quickly.

Prior knowledge. The full-threshold and fast-threshold strategies were developed at a time when our understanding of the nature of visual field loss in glaucoma was far less advanced than it is today. While these strategies used some prior knowledge, the starting level is set according to the thresholds of neighbouring locations when these are available. SITA uses prior knowledge more extensively. This has made it possible to reduce the number of presentations at certain locations.

No false positive catch trials. The SITA algorithm uses the time it takes the patient to press the response key to estimate the false positive response rate (see *Variability*, p. 37). An analysis of response times has shown that stimulus response times fall within a fairly narrow time window whilst false positive responses have a much broader range of response times, some shorter than the normal response window and some longer. By looking at the number of responses falling outside of the patient's normal response window it is possible to get an estimate of the false positive response rate.

Rate of stimulus presentation. The rate of stimulus presentations is set to a constant value in the full-threshold and fast-threshold strategies (it can be changed by the operator but in reality is rarely altered). The standard rate has to take into account slow responders and is, therefore, slower than it need be for many patients. The SITA algorithm monitors the patient's response rate and adjusts the presentation rate accordingly. In this way those patients that respond quickly will be presented with stimuli at a faster rate and complete the test in less time.

Early reports indicate that the objectives of reducing test time without loss of repeatability have been achieved (Wild *et al.*, 1999). The SITA standard test saves approximately 7 min/eye in comparison to the full-threshold strategy and its repeatability appears to be as good, if not a little better, than the full-threshold test. A surprising result is that its threshold estimates are, on average, approximately 1 dB higher than the full-threshold value, a factor which needs to be taken into account when comparing the results from the full-threshold strategy to those from SITA.

Bengtsson *et al.*, 1997 also developed a second SITA test (SITA fast) which was designed to be even faster but to have a poorer repeatability (similar to the fast-threshold strategy). This test is almost 10 minutes faster per eye than the full-threshold test and 4 minutes faster than the fast-threshold test. Its speed means that it can be used for routine testing of the visual field in optometric practice.

Variability

As mentioned earlier in this chapter, the result from any threshold strategy is subject to a certain degree of variability (this is why I have been referring to threshold estimates rather than values). This is, clearly, not an ideal situation. If the threshold estimates vary from one measurement to the next then how do you know when the visual field has got worse?

It is now recognized that there are two important parameters, which influence variability:

1. the test strategy and
2. the sensitivity at the test location (see Chapter 7, p. 101 and Chapter 2, p. 19).

Early perimetric strategies derived an estimate of subject variability termed 'fluctuation'. The fluctuation index was designed to help clinicians decide whether or not there had been any significant deterioration in the visual field. If the fluctuation was high then the clinician would view any changes in the threshold estimates with a certain amount of caution. If it were low then similar changes might be taken as evidence of real change.

To get an estimate of the fluctuation (again I use the term estimate because measures of fluctuation are themselves subject to variability) perimetric strategies repeated the threshold estimate at certain test locations. They then looked at the differences in the repeat estimates to come up with a value for the fluctuation (see Chapter 9, *Quantifying the results from static threshold strategies*, p. 122 for details of how this is calculated).

This measure of fluctuation is more correctly termed 'short-term fluctuation', the prefix 'short-term' being used to specify the type of variability that occurs within a single examination session (normally of approximately 20 minutes' duration). When looking at the results from different examinations of the same patient, the variability between sessions is found to be greater than that within a session. There is an additional component of variability, which is called 'long-term' fluctuation. Long-term fluctuation is the additional variability that can be expected to arise from one patient visit to another.

Short-term fluctuation is a global index, i.e. it gives a measure of variability which is supposed to apply to the whole visual field. We now know that variability is dependent upon sensitivity and that it cannot be accurately represented by a global value. For example, if a patient had an early arcuate defect where the sensitivity is reduced then the variability, or fluctuation, in this region of the visual field would be much greater than in the other areas of the visual field. The concept of a global index of fluctuation is no longer considered to be correct.

Total deviation and pattern deviation probability plots

Total deviation and pattern deviation probability maps take the threshold data from a visual field examination and calculate, for each test location, whether or not the threshold values are significantly different from those of a normal eye of the same age. They rely upon the perimeter having a database of threshold values from normal eyes which not only gives the average sensitivity for each test location (from which defect information is derived) but also the distribution of threshold values. Figure 3.13 helps to explain this. The two graphs in this figure represent the distribution of sensitivity values in a normal group of patients for a central and a peripheral test location. Note how they are different and that they are asymmetrical with long tails. The distribution is broader for the peripheral location, i.e. normal patients are more variable in

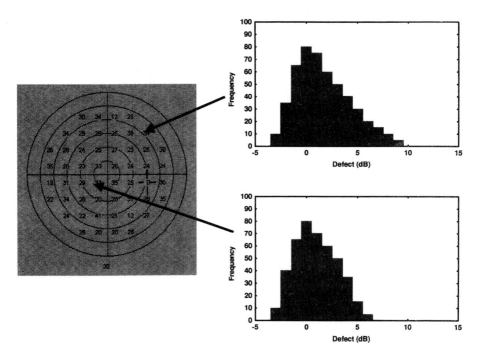

Fig. 3.13 *Distribution of thresholds at two locations in the visual field. The distribution from each test location is used to calculate total and pattern deviation probability values.*

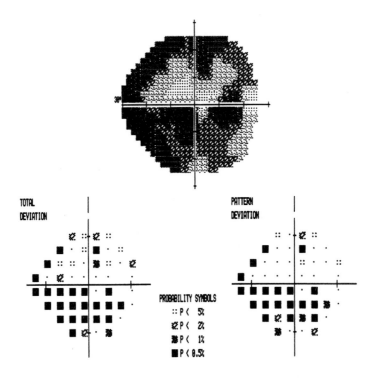

Fig. 3.14 *Grey scale printout with total and pattern deviation probability maps from Humphrey Visual Field Analyzer.*

their thresholds at this location compared to ones nearer the centre of the visual field.

The total deviation probability maps use these distributions to calculate whether the results from each location of a visual field test are within or outside of the normal range of values. The results are expressed in the standard statistical way, i.e. as being beyond the 5, 2, 1 or 0.5% level (see Figure 3.14). This simply means that there is a less than 5, 2, 1, or 0.5% chance that the measured sensitivity value comes from a normal eye.

Probability plots are very useful in that they display the significantly different points. In many ways they are similar to suprathreshold plots in that they highlight those locations which are abnormal.

Pattern deviation probability values differ from total deviation probability values in that they have been adjusted for overall shifts in sensitivity. For example, you might get a patient whose overall sensitivity is below that of a normal patient of the same age. In this case some locations may be highlighted as being abnormal on the total deviation probability map but not on the pattern deviation probability map because this map has compensated for the overall lowered sensitivity. The pattern deviation probability map takes the overall shift in intensity into account by looking at some of the most sensitive results, comparing these to the most sensitive results from normal eyes. Any difference is compensated for by simply shifting all the values either up or down. Pattern deviation probability maps will mask diffuse loss, which is a common occurrence in glaucoma (Henson *et al.*, 1999).

Catch trials

Most threshold programs include a number of catch trials that are used to estimate the false positive and false negative response rates.

False positives. On occasions the program goes through the motions of presenting a stimulus but does not actually present one. If the patient presses the button, indicating that he or she saw the non-existent stimulus, then this is classified as a false positive.

False negatives. After the program has established the threshold at a number of locations it occasionally goes back and re-presents a stimulus at an intensity

Threshold	28
Number finished	68/68
Number missed	0/68
False positives	0/2
False negatives	0/1

Fig. 3.15 *False-positive and false-negative catch trial responses are normally presented on the printout as a fraction in which the denominator represents the number of the catch trials and the numerator the number of incorrect responses.*

which is above the already established threshold. If the patient fails to respond positively to this presentation then this is classified as a false negative.

The number of catch trials and errors are normally presented in the form of a fraction, the numerator representing the number of errors while the denominator represents the number of trials (see Figure 3.15).

Many patients do not give any false positive or false negative responses. Katz and Sommer (1988) reported that 72% of patients gave no false positives and 54% no false negatives. An unexpected finding of Katz and Sommer was that the number of false negative responses increased with the extent of glaucomatous field loss. This is likely to be an artefact of the algorithm used to test for false negatives and the increased variability of responses seen in locations with reduced sensitivity.

Catch trials are intended to give the perimetrist an estimate of patient reliability. Clearly, if the patient makes a high proportion of errors then that patient's results must be viewed with a certain amount of suspicion. There are, however, no published results giving the relationship between the number of errors and reliability. In fact, two papers have questioned the value of these catch trials given that errors can exceed 20% of all catch trials (Katz and Sommer, 1988; Bickler-Bluth *et al.*, 1989). The situation is further complicated by the recent work of Vingrys and Demirel (1998), who pointed out that the precision of the catch trial estimates is very low, especially when the number of errors is relatively high. For a true false positive rate of 33% (33% chance that the patient will press the button when no stimulus is presented) estimates derived from catch trials could lie anywhere between 7 and 57% (95% confidence limits). The poor precision of the catch trial estimate is simply due to the relatively low number of catch trials within any given examination. Unfortunately, increasing them by a small amount would not result in a significant improvement. The poor precision of the catch trial estimate rather makes a mockery of the current policy of using a single cut-off value for accepting the visual field test as being 'reliable'.

The poor precision of catch trial estimates has been addressed by Olsson *et al.* (1997). They devised a technique based upon the patient's response times to perimetric stimuli. They established that patients normally respond to a stimulus within a particular response time window and then showed that the number of responses outside of the time window was proportional to their false positive rate. The advantage of looking at response times is that (1) it gives a more precise estimate and (2) it does not require any false positive trials (i.e. it shortens the examination time). This technique of estimating false positive responses has been incorporated into the SITA threshold strategy (*The dynamic strategy*, p. 35).

Conclusions

Several threshold strategies have been developed for perimetry following the original work of Bebie and Spahr. These have attempted to address some of the problems facing threshold estimates. The most recent strategies (TOP and SITA) have largely overcome the problem of extended test times. These tests still, however, show poor repeatability in cases where there is some loss of sensitivity. There is still a need for new strategies that overcome this problem.

REFERENCES

Batko K.A., Anctil J. and Anderson D.R. (1983) Detecting glaucomatous damage with the Friedmann Visual Field Analyser compared with the Goldmann perimeter and evaluation of stereoscopic photographs of the optic disk. *Am J Ophthalmol*, **95**, 435–437.

Bebie H., Fankhauser F. and Spahr J. (1976a) Static perimetry: accuracy and fluctuations. *Acta Ophthalmol*, **54**, 339–348.

Bebie H., Fankhauser F. and Spahr J. (1976b) Static perimetry: strategies. *Acta Ophthalmol*, **54**, 325–338.

Bengtsson B., Olsson J., Heijl A. and Rootzén H. (1997) A new generation of algorithms for computerised threshold perimetry, SITA. *Acta Ophthalmol*, **75**, 368–375.

Bengtsson B. and Heijl A. (1998) SITA fast, a new rapid perimetric threshold test. Description of methods and evaluation in patients with manifest and suspect glaucoma. *Acta Ophthalmol*, **76**, 431–437.

Bickler-Bluth M., Trick G.L., Kolker A.E. and Cooper D.G. (1989) Assessing the utility of reliability indices for automated visual fields. *Ophthalmol*, **96**, 616–619.

Chauhan B. (1987) PhD thesis.

De Jong D.G.M.M., Greve E.L., Baker D. and Van Den Berg T.J.T.P. (1985) Psychological factors in computer assisted perimetry; automatic and semi-automatic perimetry. *Doc Ophthalmol Proc Series*, **42**, 137–146.

Drance S.M. (1969) The early field defects in glaucoma. *Invest Ophthalmol*, **8**, 84–91.

Flammer J., Drance S.M. and Zulauf M. (1984a) Differential light threshold short and long-term fluctuations in patients with glaucoma, normal controls and patients with suspect glaucoma. *Arch Ophthalmol*, **102**, 704–706.

Flammer J., Drance S.M., Fankhauser F. and Augustiny L. (1984b) Differential light threshold in automatic static perimetry: factors influencing the short-term fluctuation. *Arch Ophthalmol*, **102**, 876–879.

Flammer J., Drance S.M. and Schultzer M. (1984c) Covariates of the long-term fluctuation of the differential light threshold. *Arch Ophthalmol*, **102**, 880–882.

Glass E., Schaumberger M. and Lachenmayr B.J. (1995) Simulations for FASTPAC and the standard 4–2 dB full-threshold strategy of the Humphrey Field Analyzer. *Invest Ophthalmol Vis Sci*, **36**, 1847–1854.

González de la Rosa M., Martinez A., Sanchez M., Mesa C., Cordoves L. and Losada M.J. (1997) Accuracy of tendency-orientated-perimetry with the Octopus 1-2-3 perimeter. In *Perimetry Update 1996/1997* (eds Wall M. and Heijl A.) Kugler, Amsterdam, pp. 119–123.

Guilford J.P. (1984) *Psychometric Methods*. Tata McGraw Hill, New Delhi.

Gutteridge I.F. (1983) The working threshold approach to Friedmann Visual Field Analyser screening. *Ophthalmic Physiol Optics*, **1**, 41–46.

Greve E.L. and Verduin W.M. (1977) Detection of early glaucomatous damage. Part 1: Visual field examination. *Doc Ophthalmol Proc Series*, **14**, 243–250.

Harrington D.O. (1976) *The Visual Fields. A Textbook and Atlas of Clinical Perimetry*. Mosby, St Louis.

Heijl A., Lindgren G. and Olsson J. (1987) Normal variability of static perimetric threshold values across the central visual field. *Arch Ophthalmol*, **105**, 1544–1549.

Henson D.B. and Anderson R. (1989) Thresholds using single and multiple stimulus presentations. In *Perimetry Update 1988/89* (ed. Heijl A.). Kugler & Ghedini, Amsterdam, pp. 191–196.

Henson D.B. and Anderson R. (1991) Threshold-related suprathreshold field testing: which is the best technique of establishing the threshold? In *Perimetry Update 1990/91* (eds Mills R. and Heijl A.). Kugler & Ghedini, Amsterdam, pp. 367–372.

Henson D.B., Artes P.H., Chaudry S.J. and Chauhan B.C. (2000) Suprathreshold perimetry: establishing the test intensity. In *Perimetry Update 1998/99* (ed. Wall M.). Kugler & Ghedini, Amsterdam, pp. 243–252.

Henson D.B., Artes P.H. and Chauhan B.C. (1999) Diffuse loss of sensitivity in early glaucoma. *Invest Ophthalmol Vis Sci*, **40**, 3147–3151.

Humphrey (1986) *The Field Analyzer Primer*. Allergan Humphrey.

Katz J. and Sommer A. (1988) Reliability indexes of automated perimetric tests. *Arch Ophthalmol*, **106**, 1252–1254.

King D., Drance S.M., Douglas G.R. and Wijsman K. (1986) The detection of paracentral scotomas with varying grids in computed perimetry. *Arch Ophthalmol*, **104**, 524–525.

Olsson J., Bengtsson B., Heijl A. and Rootzen H. (1997) An improved method to estimate frequency of false positive answers in computerized perimetry. *Acta Ophthalmol*, **75**, 18–183.

Spahr J. (1975) Optimization of the presentation pattern in automated static perimetry. *Vis Res*, **15**, 1275–1281.

Vingrys A.J. and Demirel S. (1998) False response monitoring during automated perimetry. *Optom Vis Sci*, **75**, 513–517.

Weber J. and Rau S. (1992) The properties of Perimetric thresholds in normal and glaucomatous eyes. *Germ J Ophthalmol*, **1**, 79–85.

Wild J.M., Pacey I.E., Hancock S.A. and Cunliffe I.A. (1999) Between-algorithm, between-individual differences in normal perimetric sensitivity: full threshold, FASTPAC and SITA. *Invest Ophthalmol Vis Sci*, **40**, 1152–61.

4 Alternative strategies for examining the visual field

INTRODUCTION

The previous chapter dealt with the main examination strategies currently being used to examine the visual field. This chapter goes on to describe six additional strategies which are all commercially available:

- Blue-on-yellow perimetry.
- High pass resolution perimetry.
- Frequency doubling perimetry.
- Confrontation tests.
- Oculokinetic perimetry.
- Amsler charts.

Two of these, confrontation and oculokinetic perimetry, are designed for quick screening of the visual field when conventional field testing equipment is not available. The Amsler chart is designed to assess the central 10 degrees of the visual field while the other techniques have all been designed to increase test sensitivity and/or ease of use.

For a review of alternative visual function tests in glaucoma (such as electrophysiology) the reader is referred to Stewart and Chauhan (1995).

BLUE–YELLOW PERIMETRY

For a number of years it has been recognized that patients with glaucoma often have an associated colour vision defect in which their sensitivity to blue light is reduced. This observation led researchers to question whether or not the blue sensitive mechanism was more susceptible to glaucomatous damage and whether or not a perimeter that specifically targeted the blue mechanism might not be more sensitive than those that use the conventional white stimuli.

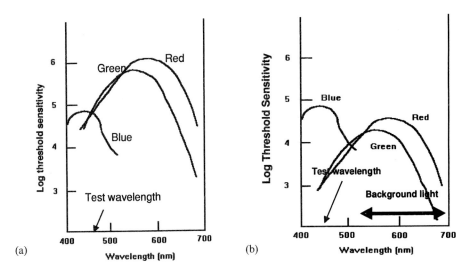

Fig. 4.1 *The sensitivity of the 3-colour vision mechanism (a) under normal conditions and (b) after adaptation to a yellow light. Note how the adaptation to the yellow light selectively attenuates the red and green mechanisms and increases the exposure of the blue mechanism.*

A problem encountered when trying to test the blue mechanism is the relatively low sensitivity of blue cones, even at short wavelengths (see Figure 4.1a). At 440 nm the blue sensitive cones are only marginally more sensitive than the red and green cones. Selective damage to the blue cones would have relatively little effect upon sensitivity as the red and green cones would simply step in once the blue cone sensitivity dropped below that of the other receptors. To overcome this problem the red and green cones are de-sensitized by adapting the eye to a yellow light. Figure 4.1(b) shows the sensitivity of the three receptors after adaptation. The blue cones are now more exposed at the 440 nm wavelength. The extent of exposure is important. If you consider that any damage to the blue cones mechanism is likely to lower its sensitivity you can see from this figure just how much loss can be tolerated before the red and green receptors again become the most sensitive (approximately 1.5 log units).

Blue–yellow perimetry is an option in both the 600 and 700 series of Humphrey Visual Field Analyzers. This instrument uses a 440 nm filter for its stimulus and an OG530 (Schott) for background. The background luminance is much brighter than for white-on-white perimetry ($100\,cd^2$ rather than 10) and the standard stimulus is larger, Goldmann V rather than III.

There have been a number of studies that have evaluated the potential of blue–yellow perimetry. One of the best of these was a five-year longitudinal study conducted by Johnson *et al.* (1993). They demonstrated that blue–yellow defects precede those for white-on-white perimetry, blue–yellow defects predict which ocular hypertensive patients will develop white-on-white defects and blue–yellow defects are, on average, larger than those for white-on-white perimetry.

Despite being more sensitive than white-on-white perimetry and readily available for routine clinical practice blue–yellow perimetry has not been widely adopted. There are a number of possible reasons for this.

1. The effect of lens opacities. Blue–yellow perimetry is particularly sensitive to lens opacities. The yellowing of the crystalline lens, a common occurrence in the elderly, selectively absorbs blue light and lowers the sensitivity to blue stimuli. There are a number of ways of compensating for lens absorption but these all involve an additional measure that can be time consuming.

2. Patients dislike the technique, even more so than the standard white-on-white threshold techniques.

3. There is an increase in the variability of the responses. This is, partially, compensated for by the use of a larger stimulus. It is the signal to noise ratio that is important in perimetry. If the noise level is higher then there needs to be an increase in the signal just to maintain the same discriminatory power.

4. The main value of the technique, increased sensitivity, is only pertinent to a small percentage of patients attending for a visual field examination. Most patients seen in a glaucoma clinic already have visual field loss with white-on-white perimetry. There have been no studies demonstrating that blue–yellow perimetry is more sensitive at detecting progressive loss.

HIGH PASS RESOLUTION PERIMETRY

Frisen (1987) has developed a new form of perimetry based upon the resolution of ring-shaped targets of varying size (see Figure 4.2). The targets are presented on a monitor whose mean background luminance is $20 \, cd/m^2$. The luminance inside each ring target is the same as the background while the core of the ring is brighter and its inner and outer edges darker. The overall intensity profile of the ring is such that when it cannot be resolved it cannot be detected. In the words of Frisen it 'melts, imperceptibly into the background'.

The task of the patient is similar to that of conventional static perimetry. A ring of predetermined size is presented (presentation time 165 msec) at a given position within the visual field and the patient asked

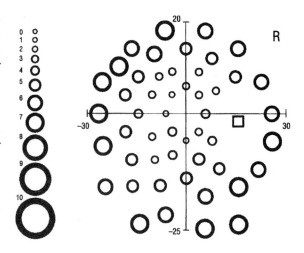

Fig. 4.3 *Example of the output from a patient with a normal visual field measured with high pass resolution perimetry. Note the larger ring size towards the periphery representing the lower resolution in the peripheral field.*

to respond with a key press whenever it is seen. A repetitive bracketing strategy (one reversal) is used to establish the minimum resolvable ring size at a series of 50 retinal locations within the central 30 degrees (see Figure 4.3).

High pass resolution perimetry has good sensitivity and specificity when compared to conventional (white-on-white) full-threshold perimetry (Martinez *et al.*, 1995). It has also been shown to have threshold variability that is independent of sensitivity and can detect progressive loss earlier than conventional perimetry (Chauhan *et al.*, 1999).

High pass resolution perimetry is considerably faster than conventional perimetry, taking on average only 5.5 minutes to test 50 test locations (conventional full-threshold perimetry takes more than twice as long. The shorter test time is one of the reasons that this test is more acceptable to patients.

On the negative side the technique is sensitive to blur, either refractive or due to media changes, unable to measure defect depth within small circumscribed lesions, and is unable to detect scotoma whose size is less than the local liminal test target. With the current monitor technology there is also a relatively small dynamic range of stimuli which limits the test ability to monitor loss in patients who have advanced defects but some important residual sensitivity.

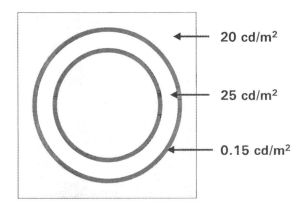

Fig. 4.2 *Ring stimulus used in high pass resolution perimetry.*

20 cd/m²

25 cd/m²

0.15 cd/m²

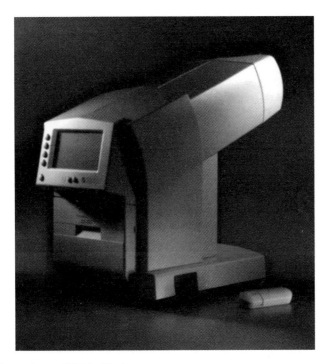

Fig. 4.4 *Frequency doubling perimeter (Welch Allen).*

FREQUENCY DOUBLING PERIMETRY

Despite all the developments in perimetry over the past few years, there is still a pressing need for a quick and simple screening/early detection test which combines ease of use with high sensitivity and specificity. While a number of perimeters incorporate screening/fast programmes the nature of these instruments makes them less than ideal for screening where portability, independence of both refractive error and room illumination are important design parameters.

A new visual field screener/analyser – the frequency doubling perimeter – has recently been developed by Welch Allen (distributed by Zeiss) (see Figure 4.4). The stimulus parameters used within this instrument are based upon an illusion known as frequency doubling (Kelly, 1966), in which an alternating sinusoidal grating of low spatial frequency (>4 cpd) appears, at certain temporal frequencies (>15 Hz), to have twice as many lines. This illusion, the frequency doubling illusion, is believed to be mediated by the magnocellular (M-cell) pathway and in particular by the large fibre diameter M_y ganglion cells which constitute 1.5–2.5% of all retinal ganglion cells.

Why is this important? Well an analysis of the ganglion cell fibre loss associated with glaucoma has led to the development of a number of theories. One theory is that there is selective loss of magnocellular fibres during the early stages of this condition. Another is that there is selective loss of large diameter axons and a third is that mechanisms with little redundancy (sparse representation) are likely to show losses earlier than those with greater redundancy. As the frequency doubling illusion is believed to be based upon large diameter magnocellular fibres which are sparsely represented, a screening test based upon this illusion should, according to all these theories, be particularly sensitive to early glaucomatous loss.

While the frequency doubling perimeter uses the appropriate spatial and temporal frequencies for the frequency doubling illusion the task presented to the patient is one of contrast sensitivity, i.e. the patient is being asked when he can detect the appearance of a target in the peripheral field not when he sees the frequency doubling illusion. The name of the instrument is, therefore, somewhat inappropriate and its theoretical basis somewhat suspect.

While early work on frequency doubling perimetry was conducted by Maddess, the currently manufactured instrument is based upon the results of Johnson and Samuels (1997), who refined the psychophysical strategy and established the optimal number of test locations. The current instrument, which uses a modified binary search strategy and 17 test locations, has been reported to have a sensitivity of 93% and a specificity of 100%. Average test time was 5 minutes 14 seconds. A later report (Johnson *et al.*, 1997) gave similar findings from a much larger population. There are currently no published reports on the screening strategy incorporated in this instrument, which is claimed to take less than 1 minute per eye.

The frequency doubling perimeter has many attractive characteristics for glaucoma screening. It is a small, self-contained, portable instrument that is not sensitive to background illumination levels. It does not require a corrective lens for refractive errors (results are reported to be independent of refractive error up to $+/-7.00\,D$). It is quick and purported to have both high sensitivity and specificity.

AMSLER CHARTS

Many perimetric instruments have relatively few stimuli within the central 10 degrees and it is, therefore, often difficult, if not impossible, to accurately map central defects. One solution to this problem is to use Amsler charts. These were first introduced in 1947 (Amsler, 1947, 1953) to assist in the detection of early macular disease. Their use has been widened today to include the detection of all conditions affecting the central 10 degrees of the visual field.

The charts consist of a series of cards, each with a central fixation point and a regular pattern of markings. The most widely used chart has a regular 1 degree square matrix of white lines on a black background (see Figure 4.5).

The patient's task is to fixate the centre of the chart, which is held at 30 cm from the eye, and to describe, or draw (on a separate recording chart) where the lines are missing or distorted. Research has shown that these areas coincide with regions of retinal disturbance.

The attractions of this test are its simplicity and high sensitivity. Klein *et al.* (1974) and Natsikos and Dean Hart (1980) both reported that the vast majority of patients with central serous retinopathy reported

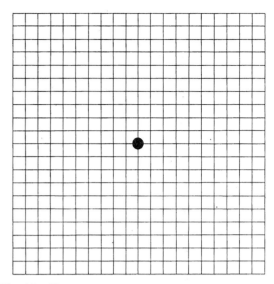

Fig. 4.5   *The appearance of the most widely used Amsler chart. The lines are white on a black background.*

changes in the appearance of the Amsler charts and Wall and Sadun (1986) have demonstrated that, in patients with optic neuropathy, Amsler testing is both considerably faster and more sensitive than both conventional tangent screen examination or full-threshold perimetry. This finding reflects the relative paucity of central stimuli in most perimetric strategies.

CONFRONTATION TEST

The confrontation test is a relatively crude technique to screen for the presence of unsuspected field defects. It is often included as part of a routine eye examination when no formal examination of the visual field is called for.

There are two different strategies for conducting a confrontation test. The first I have called the 'traditional strategy' simply because it is currently the most widely practised version. The second, is the 'comparison strategy'.

Traditional confrontation strategy

The patient, with one eye occluded, is asked to fixate either the eye or nose of the examiner who sits opposite within a metre's distance. The examiner then introduces fingers or hand-held targets into the patient's field from the periphery in a plane approximately equidistant from the patient and practitioner. The patient is asked to report when he or she can see the target or, in the case where different numbers of fingers are being held up, how many fingers can be seen. The test is a comparison of the practitioner's visual field with that of the patient to establish whether or not there is any significant constriction or a scotoma. A variant of this technique, kinetic boundary testing, involves moving the stimulus along an arc from behind the patient's head. This variant allows the practitioner to estimate the peripheral limits for the target, which will often extend beyond the practitioner's reach with the traditional test. It is not uncommon for practitioners to use a combination of these two tests when examining a patient.

Table 4.1 Sensitivity of the confrontation test to different types of pathology

Defect type	Number	Sensitivity (%)
Altitudinal	7	100
Central/centrocecal	5	100
Monocular hemianopia	3	67
Constriction	9	44
Paracentral	3	22
Arcuate	36	22
Patchy defects	27	7
Junctional scotoma	4	75
Homonymous hemianopia	23	74
Bitemporal hemianopia	10	40

Source: Johnson and Baloh, 1988.

Suprathreshold comparison strategy

In this situation a suprathreshold target, one that is bright enough to be easily seen, is presented in the four different quadrants and the patient asked if it appears brighter or dimmer in any of the quadrants. If a coloured target is used then they would be asked if the colour appears different. This strategy is fundamentally different to the traditional strategy in that patients are being asked to compare the appearance of the target as it is transferred from one quadrant to another rather than simply reporting whether or not they can see it.

A variant of this type of test, the Red Dot Test, has been developed by Mutlukan and Cullen (1991). The test is composed of a card with a ring of eight red dots and a central black fixation point. When held at 30 cm the red dots fall at an eccentricity of 25 degrees. The patient's task is to look at the fixation point and to count the number of red dots. Missing dots implies the presence of an absolute scotoma. The patient is also asked if any of the dots appear washed out in order to detect relative scotoma. In a comparison with the Bjerrum screen, Mutlukan and Cullen have demonstrated that the test can detect a significant number of visual field defects.

Sensitivity of confrontation tests

Measuring the sensitivity of confrontation tests poses a number of problems. The first is the exact nature of the confrontation test. While two different techniques have been described, clinicians seem to develop their own particular way of performing this test, which they believe to be optimal often with little if any supportive data. A second problem is the choice of validating criteria. What is the confrontation test being compared to? Some clinicians compare it to routine kinetic tests, while others have compared it to a full-threshold static test. Clearly if the confrontation test is compared to a test with a high sensitivity then it will not appear as sensitive as it would be if compared to a test of low sensitivity. A third problem relates to the population of field defects used in the evaluation. If this only includes patients with severe visual field loss then the confrontation test will again appear more sensitive than if the sample included a lot of subtle defects.

Having presented you with all the problems associated with the evaluation of confrontation tests, it is now time to present you with some results. Table 4.1 gives some of the results from a study by Johnson and Baloh (1988) in which a confrontation test was compared with a full-threshold static test (76 test points in the central 30 degrees). It is interesting to note that Johnson and Baloh found the confrontation test to be most sensitive to altitudinal, centrocecal and pathway defects, with the exception of bitemporal hemianopia, and that its sensitivity to glaucoma-type defects (paracentral and arcuate) is low.

Similar results were obtained by Trobe *et al.* (1980), who in addition to reporting on the overall sensitivity of confrontation tests also compared the traditional technique, which involved finger counting, with a colour comparison technique. They found the finger counting technique to be less sensitive than the colour comparison technique, particularly at detecting chiasmal hemianopic defects. An excellent and comprehensive review of confrontation tests has been published by Elliott *et al.* (1997).

OCULOKINETIC PERIMETRY

Oculokinetic perimetry is, contrary to what the name might imply, a form of static perimetry. It derives its name from the fact that the patient's eye moves to different fixation points while the test stimulus remains stationary. The test has been developed by Damato (1985), who has promoted it as a community based screening test for glaucoma. Damato recognized

that the complexity of many perimetric tests is a disincentive to routine visual field screening, with the result that clinicians are often reluctant to request a visual field examination unless the patient meets certain preconditions. Given that the other types of screening tests for glaucoma (measurement of the intraocular pressure and optic nerve head evaluation) have a relatively low sensitivity, there is a danger that extensive field loss can go undetected. It is envisaged that the charts will be distributed to the relatives of patients with glaucoma and to community health care workers.

In practice, the patient views a white tangent screen on which a series of numbers are printed surrounding a central black test stimulus (see Figure 4.6). The

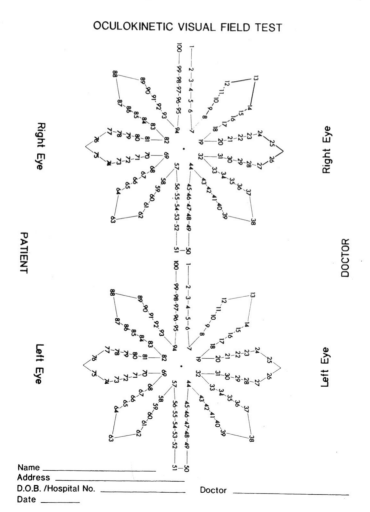

Fig. 4.6   *One of the Oculokinetic visual field tests.*

patient's task is to look at each of the numbers in sequence and to note whether or not they can see the central stimulus. They then mark any location where the stimulus could not be seen.

Several different versions of this test have been developed (see Harper, 1991, for a review); the most promising is a hand-held version with just 23 test locations (Damato *et al.*, 1990).

An important property of any screening test is its specificity. If this is not high then any benefits accruing from a rapid screening test may be totally negated by the large number of false positives. With conventional perimeters a screening failure is normally subjected to further visual field examination to establish whether any failure is a true or false positive. This can be done by either extending the number of stimuli presented, testing at higher intensities or running a second, non-screening, programme. The oculokinetic test does not, currently, allow for further investigation and is, therefore, likely to lead to a greater number of false positives.

The speed of the oculokinetic test is approximately the same as that of a multiple stimulus suprathreshold test of equivalent number of stimuli.

In conclusion, this type of test does not seem to offer the clinician with access to conventional field screening instruments/programmes any additional benefits. However, it is of value when such access is not available.

REFERENCES

Amsler M. (1947) L'examen qualitatif de la fonction maculaire. *Ophthalmologica*, **114**, 248–261.

Amsler M. (1953) Earliest symptoms of disease of the macular. *Br J Ophthalmol*, **37**, 521–537.

Chauhan B.C., House P.H., McCormick T.A. and LeBlanc R.P. (1999) Comparison of conventional and high-pass resolution perimetry in a prospective study of patients with glaucoma and healthy controls. *Arch Ophthalmol*, **117**, 24–33.

Damato B.E. (1985) A simple field test for use in the community. *Br J Ophthalmol*, **69**, 927–931.

Damato B.E., Chyla J., McClure E., Jay J. and Allan D. (1990) A hand-held OKP chart for the screening of glaucoma: Preliminary evaluation. *Eye*, **4**, 632–637.

Elliott D.B., North I. and Flanagan J. (1997) Confrontation visual field tests. *Ophthal Physiol Optics*, **17**, Suppl. 2, pp. S17–S24.

Frisen L. (1987) A computer-graphics visual field screener using high-pass spatial frequency resolution and multiple feedback devices. *Doc Ophthalmol Proc Series*, **49**, 441–446.

Harper R. (1991) Oculo-kinetic perimetry: a review. *Optician* 22 February, pp. 13, 15, 17, 36–38.

Johnson C.A. and Samuels S.J. (1997) Screening for glaucomatous visual field loss with frequency-doubling perimetry. *Invest Ophthalmol Vis Sci*, **38**, 413–425.

Johnson C.A., Adams A.J. and Casson E.J. (1993) Blue-on-yellow perimetry: a five-year overview. In *Perimetry Update 1992/1993* (ed. Mills R.P.). Kugler & Ghedini, Amsterdam, pp. 459–465.

Johnson C.A., Cello K.E., Nelson-Quigg J.M. and Demirel S. (1997) Performance of frequency doubling perimetry for detecting various levels of glaucomatous visual field loss. ARVO Abs. *Invest Ophthalmol Vis Sci*, **38**, S200.

Johnson L.N. and Baloh F. G. (1989) Confrontation visual field test in comparison with automated perimetry. In *Perimetry Update 1988/89* (ed. Heijl A.). Kugler & Ghedini, Amsterdam, pp 85–90.

Kelly D.H. (1966) Frequency doubling in visual responses. *J Opt Soc Am A*, **56**, 1628–1633.

Klein M.L., Van Buskirk M., Friedmann E., Gragoudas E. and Chandra S. (1974) Experience with non-treatment of central serous retinopathy. *Arch Ophthalmol*, **91**, 247–250.

Maddess T., Goldberg I., Dobinson J., Wine S. and James A.C. (1995) Clinical trials of the frequency doubled illusions an indicator of glaucoma. *ARVO Abs Invest Ophthalmol Vis Sci*, **35**, 335.

Martinez G.A., Sample P.A. and Weinreb R.N. (1995) Comparison of high-pass resolution perimetry and standard automated perimetry in glaucoma. *Am J Ophthalmol*, **119**, 195–201.

Mutlukan E. and Cullen J.F. (1991) Red colour comparison perimetry chart in neuro-ophthalmological examination. *Eye*, **5**, 352–361.

Natsikos V.E. and Dean Hart J.C. (1980) Static perimetry and Amsler chart changes in patients with idiopathic central serous retinopathy. *Acta Ophthalmol*, **58**, 908–917.

Stewart W.C. and Chauhan B.C. (1995) Newer visual function tests in the evaluation of glaucoma. *Surv Ophthalmol*, **40**, 119–135.

Trobe J.D., Acosta P.C., Krischer J.P. and Trick G.L. (1980) Confrontation visual field techniques in the detection of anterior visual pathway lesions. *Ann Neurol*, **10**, 28–34.

Wall M. and Sadun A.A. (1986) Threshold Amsler grid testing. *Arch Ophthalmol*, **104**, 520–523.

5 Extraneous factors which affect the visual field

INTRODUCTION

One of the most frustrating moments for the perimetrist is when he or she realizes, at the end of an exhaustive examination, that they forgot to include a refractive correction or that they forgot to tell the patient to keep their eye wide open. What makes matters even worse is that such omissions can often simulate the types of field loss found in ocular pathologies. What does the perimetrist do? Go through the whole procedure again? Does the neglected factor really have a significant effect upon the results?

In this chapter, those annoying little parameters that all too often have a significant effect upon the results are going to be exposed. So at the end of this chapter you will at least know what the likely effects of any omission will be, even if you do have to repeat the whole examination.

Some of the parameters that will be discussed can be considered as artefacts. They are caused by obstacles, such as the spectacle frame or eyelashes, obscuring the visual field. Others are due to changes in the eye, such as variations in pupil size and media transparency.

THE EFFECT OF AGE UPON THE VISUAL FIELD

While age is often associated with a maturity of thought, it unfortunately also coincides with less desirable effects, one of which is a gradual reduction in the eye's sensitivity. The cause of this loss has been variously ascribed to factors such as:

1. Changes in pupil size (see later section in this chapter).

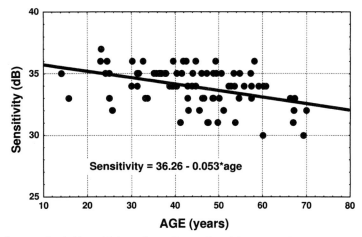

Fig. 5.1 *Relationship between threshold sensitivity and age. Data collected from a population of 'normal' patients with the Henson Pro perimeter.*

2. Changes in the transmission of the ocular media (particularly the lens).
3. Changes in the sensitivity of the retina and visual pathways.

A paper by Johnson *et al.* (1989) concludes that the majority of this loss is due to changes in the sensitivity of the retina and visual pathways, although, clearly, other factors such as media transparency will also have an effect.

Age changes and kinetic perimetry

In kinetic perimetry this age-related loss in sensitivity, which can be thought of as a slight sinking of the island of vision, results in a contraction of the isopters. Drance *et al.* (1967) were among the first researchers to quantify the extent of this loss. They demonstrated that the area (mm^2 on visual field chart) enclosed by the I-2 isopter on the Goldmann bowl perimeter decreased linearly with age and that the rate of change could be fitted by the equation:

$$\text{Area} = 4045 - 30.74 \times (\text{age in years})$$

A similar result was found by both Hart and Becker (1977) and by Williams (1983), although in both cases they found the rate of decline and the y-intercept to be greater than that reported by Drance *et al.* (1967). Williams suggests that these differences could be accounted for on the basis of different perimetric techniques, including the nature of the instructions given to the patient. It should be recalled that with kinetic perimetry the results are heavily influenced by the perimetric technique.

Age changes and static perimetry

In static perimetry age-related loss manifests itself as a lowering of the estimated thresholds. The majority of researchers who have investigated this problem have concluded that there is a linear relationship between the static threshold and age, the sensitivity declining at a rate of between 0.4 and 0.8 dB per decade (Brenton and Phelps, 1986; Haas *et al.*, 1986; Jaffe *et al.*, 1986; Heijl *et al.*, 1987) (see Figure 5.1). In an analysis of how age affects a whole series of different visual functions, Johnson and Choy (1987) demonstrated that most functions, rather than having a constant rate of decline, appeared to have two separate stages. In people under the age of 50 the decline with age was only slight, while for those over the age of 50 it was much faster.

Threshold variability and age

It appears that not only does the rate of sensitivity loss increase with age but also the spread of results within any particular age group. In the older age groups there is a greater spread of values; some patients have sensitivities that are only slightly below those of much younger patients while others show quite marked sensitivity losses. This finding could simply be a reflection of the increased variability in media transmission that is known to occur with age. The increased spread of results has important practical implication. It means that the use of age settings in suprathreshold tests and age-corrected normal values in full threshold tests are subject to larger errors in the older age groups. Thus, while a reduction in the index 'mean defect' (see Chapter 9 for a definition of this index) might make the perimetrist suspicious in a young person, it might merely indicate some early lens changes in an older patient.

Age changes and eccentricity

Several researchers have investigated whether these age-related changes are constant across the whole visual field or whether they vary with eccentricity. The majority report that the decline is greater at an eccentricity of 30 degrees (the limit of the area tested in these studies) than it is at the centre of the visual field (Hass *et al.*, 1986; Jaffe *et al.*, 1986; Heijl *et al.*, 1987). In other words, the hill of vision not only sinks with age but also gets steeper. A conflicting view is held by Brenton and Phelps (1986), who reported no significant difference between the rates of decline at the centre of the visual field and at an eccentricity of 30 degrees. They suggested that some of the apparent discrepancy between their findings and those of other researchers might be explained on the basis of the way in which the data was collected. The Humphrey and Octopus instruments, which were used in all of the previously cited studies, establish the threshold of the peripheral points last. The effects of fatigue, which would generally result in a reduced sensitivity (see p. 60) would be greater at the peripheral points.

It is also of interest to note that cataracts normally steepen the sensitivity profile (see p. 61) and that the increasing occurrence of cataracts in the older age groups may, in part, explain why the gradient of sensitivity steepens with age.

PUPIL SIZE

The pupil of the eye acts very much like the aperture stop on a camera. It controls the amount of light reaching the retina and, as a result, the perimetric thresholds.

When considering the effects of pupil size upon the visual field the perimetrist should bear in mind the extreme variations in pupil diameter that can result from different types of medication. Pilocarpine, which is prescribed to lower the intra-ocular pressure in patients with glaucoma, causes a marked miosis, the pupil diameter usually being less than 2 mm.

It is not uncommon for the perimetrist to be presented with a follow-up case to evaluate in which a miotic drug, like pilocarpine, has been prescribed since the last visual field measurement. In such situations it is important that the perimetrist knows what the likely effects of pupil constriction are so that he or she can evaluate whether any changes are the result of the miosis or more sinister changes in the visual field.

The important thing to realize about pupil constriction is that it dims both the intensity of the stimulus and that of the background. The contrast of the stimulus, which is defined as the ratio of the stimulus increment to its background ($\Delta I/I$), is not affected by alterations in pupil size.

Pupil size and background intensity

The ability to detect a stimulus depends largely upon its contrast. At high photopic levels, the relationship between contrast and thresholds is described by the Weber–Fechner law, which states that $\Delta I/I$ = constant, where I is the intensity of the background and ΔI is the difference in intensity between the stimulus and the background. At photopic levels, therefore, pupil miosis should have little if any effect upon detection.

As the luminance falls to the lower photopic/upper mesopic levels so this convenient relationship between contrast and detection breaks down (see Chapter 2 for more details on the relationship between ΔI and I). At these intensity levels any change in the background intensity I, such as that brought about by pupil constriction, will require a brighter stimulus to reach threshold values.

In the Goldmann instrument, and those that use Goldmann equivalent background levels (32.5 asb), where the background intensity is comparatively high, the effect of changes in pupil size is slight. Isopter area shows a small reduction with miosis, as do threshold levels. Lindenmuth *et al.* (1989) using the Humphrey Visual Field Analyzer (which uses Goldmann equivalent levels of background illumination) found an average sensitivity loss of only 0.67 dB when they instilled pilocarpine to constrict the pupil

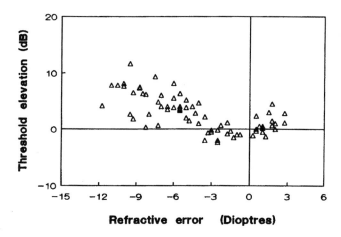

Fig. 5.2 *The effect of defocus upon threshold sensitivity. Data collected with Henson CFA3000.*

(see also Heuer *et al.*, 1989). This reduction in sensitivity is much less than would be predicted from a simple measurement of pupil area. In Lindenmuth *et al.'s* (1989) study the mean pupil area reduced from 16.29 mm^2 to 4.32 mm^2, an approximate four-fold drop, which would be equivalent to 6 dB. The fact that the sensitivity reduced by only 0.67 dB demonstrates how closely the visual system follows the Weber–Fechner law at this background luminance. Edgar *et al.* (1999), in a group of young volunteers whose pupil area changed from 23.67 mm^2 to 4.01 mm^2, reported a slightly larger effect (2 dB) whilst studies conducted on an older population of patients with glaucomatous visual field defect gave a reduction of 1.49 dB (Webster *et al.*, 1993).

The breakdown of the Weber–Fechner law at low background luminances means that instruments with lower background luminances, such as the Friedmann, Henson, Octopus 101 and Tubinger, will be more sensitive to changes in pupil size.

Cataract is a confounding factor to the effects of pupil constriction. Patients with some degree of cataract and large pupils can often 'look around' their opacities. When their pupils are constricted they can lose this ability and, as a result, show considerable shifts in their perimetric thresholds.

Pupil size and eccentricity

Before leaving this subject there is one last point to mention. The effect of pupil constriction has been reported to vary with eccentricity. Wood *et al.* (1988) have shown that the effects of pupil constriction are much greater in the periphery than in the centre of the visual field. They also noted an overall increase in the variability of threshold measures with miosis.

REFRACTIVE ERROR AND DEFOCUS

The correction of refractive errors is one of the biggest bugbears in perimetry. If you don't correct refractive errors then you get errors due to defocus and if you do correct them you get lens rim artefacts.

The major effect of defocus is to spread the target's retinal image over a larger area. This changes the luminance gradient at the edge of the target and, for small stimuli, reduces the luminance at the centre of the target. Blurring decreases the strength of the stimulus (Henson and Morris, 1993) (see Figure 5.2).

When considering the correction of refractive error in perimetry it is important to remember that refractive error changes with eccentricity (Millodot, 1981). Correcting the refractive error at the fovea does not necessarily mean that the peripheral errors are corrected for. In fact, as the predominant refractive change with eccentricity is an increase in astigmatism (oblique astigmatism), residual peripheral errors are the norm rather than the exception. The correction of the foveal refractive error is, however, important as it aids fixation and reduces accommodative fluctuation. Patients find it very difficult to keep their eye still when they are told to look at a large blurred target.

Refractive error and stimulus size

Small stimuli are more sensitive to defocus than large ones (Sloan, 1960; Atchinson, 1987). Results from Goldmann perimetry show that for stimulus size I (which subtends 7 minutes of arc) the effect of 5.00 D of simulated hyperopic blur reduces the central sensitivity by approximately 12 dB. For the frequently used size III stimulus (30 min of arc), the same blur reduces sensitivity by 6 dB, while with stimulus V (120 min of arc) the effect is less than 3 dB.

Refractive error and eccentricity

The effects of defocus are also dependent upon the eccentricity of the target. The more eccentric the target, the less it is affected by defocus. At 30 degrees from the centre of the field, 5.00 D of simulated hyperopia reduces the sensitivity by approximately 8, 4 and 3 dB respectively for stimuli I, III and V on the Goldmann perimeter (Atchinson, 1987). Similar results have been reported with the Octopus perimeter using a Goldmann III equivalent target (Benedetto and Cyrlin, 1985).

Refractive error and inter-patient variability

The effects of defocus appear to vary from one patient to another (Atchinson, 1987). While some patients may show a marked response at certain eccentricities, others will show practically no response. Part of this variability may be explained by the variations in the peripheral refractive error. Some patients' peripheral errors may move in the positive direction while others move in a negative direction (Millodot, 1981).

Practical implications relating to defocus
Threshold measuring techniques
It is clear from the above, that even small refractive errors can have a significant effect upon perimetric thresholds, particularly when small stimuli are used. To obtain as reliable and consistent data as possible refractive errors as small as 1.00 D should be corrected.

Suprathreshold screening tests
With suprathreshold strategies it may be possible to compensate for small amounts of blur when selecting the test intensity. If the effect of defocus is to produce an overall reduction in sensitivity then the intensity of the test stimuli can be increased to give a reliable

Table 5.1 Recommended corrective lens addition for different testing distances

Age (yr)	Testing distance (cm)			
	25	33	50	100
40–44	1.50			
45–49	2.00	1.00		
50–54	2.50	1.50		
55–59	3.00	2.00	1.00	
60–64	3.50	2.50	1.50	
>64	4.00	3.00	2.00	1.00

Source: Based on data of Millodot and Millodot, 1988

measure of any focal loss. Such an adjustment would automatically be incorporated in a threshold related test (see Chapter 4 on different suprathreshold strategies). There is no published data on the effect of blur upon the detection of visual field defects. Until such data exist, it is better to be cautious and correct for refractive errors in excess of 1.00 D.

Refractive error and presbyopia

As many patients undergoing a visual field examination will be presbyopic, the correction should include an adjustment for near vision. Table 5.1 gives recommended additions for different testing distances.

CORRECTING LENS ARTEFACT

While, as outlined in the previous section, it is important to use a correcting lens when examining the visual field, the diameter of standard trial case lenses makes them prone to produce a correcting lens rim artefact (see Figure 5.3).

The defect normally occurs at the edge of the central field, at an eccentricity of 25–30 degrees, and can mimic the appearance of a nerve fibre defect.

Lens rim artefacts are more common in the elderly (Zalta, 1989), presumably because their deep set eyes make it difficult to get the lens close enough to their eyes, although it could also be due to the fact that they fidget more. These artefacts are also more common in patients with hyperopia, particularly those with lens powers over +6.00 D, in which the incidence of artefacts reaches nearly 20%.

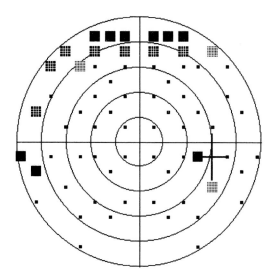

Fig. 5.3 *Lens rim artefact.*

Lens rim artefacts and test strategy

Lens rim artefacts are more frequently encountered in automated, as opposed to manual and semi-automated, strategies. The most likely explanation for this is that in manual and semi-automated strategies the perimetrist recognizes when the lens rim is causing problems and corrects for it by re-instructing the patient. In automated perimetry the results are collected in a pre-programmed manner and then analysed at the end of the test. By the time the perimetrist recognizes that a problem may exist the data have already been collected and the test completed.

The incidence of correcting lens artefact with the automated Humphrey Visual Field Analyzer has been estimated to be 10.4% in a retrospective study and 6.2% in a prospective study in which perimetrists were educated about the occurrence of this artefact and instructed to take extra care in the positioning of the patient with respect to the correcting lens (Zalta, 1989).

Methods of correcting refractive errors
Patient's own prescription

Whenever possible use the patient's own spectacle correction as this usually gives a larger field of view then the equivalent prescription in trial lens form. It is also, hopefully, more comfortable. Of course, when using the patient's own prescription you must ensure that it is single vision (not bifocal, multifocal or varifocal) and that it is appropriate for the testing distance (see Table 5.1). Perimetrists should be aware that many of the varifocal lenses look like single vision lenses. The best way to find out whether they are varifocal or single vision is to ask the patient.

Ready-glazed spectacles

An alternative is to use sets of ready-glazed spectacle frames. This technique has a lot to commend it although it will need a large number of frames to cover the necessary range of corrections.

Perimetric lens set

One of the best solutions is to use a specially designed perimetric lens set. Henson and Earlam (1995) have developed a perimetric lens set that uses a trail frame, worn by the patient, rather than a lens holder fixed to the perimeter. Anyone who has conducted a fair number of perimetric examinations knows that patients often move during the examination. When the correcting lens is attached to the perimeter this type of movement results in lens misalignment and reductions in the field of view. Attaching the lens to a trail frame worn by the patient overcomes this problem as the lens moves with the patient. The perimetric lens set developed by Henson and Earlam (see Figure 5.4) also uses large diameter lenses which give a large field of view (greater than 48 degrees in all directions). It also incorporates an occluder, thereby doing away with the uncomfortable clip and elasticised strap occluders that often irritate the patient and distract their attention during the examination.

Trial case lenses

If neither of the above solutions is available and you are forced to use a trail lens set then make sure you have large diameter trial case lenses (reduced aperture lenses are excellent for simulating tunnel vision). The lenses must be carefully aligned and the patient instructed to keep their eye as close as possible to the lens. When a suspect defect is found, this region of the field should be re-examined with the correcting lens removed. If the defect disappears then it can be safely assumed that it was due to the correcting lens.

EYELID, EYELASHES AND EYEBROW

Droopy eyelids or prominent eyelashes can result in an apparent loss of the superior peripheral field (see

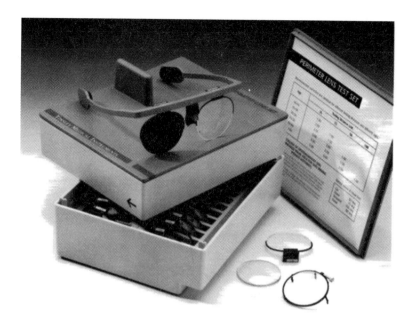

Fig. 5.4 *Perimetric lens set.*

Figure 5.5). This problem is more apparent in patients with prominent brows and deeply set eyes. It can also result from the patient being improperly positioned at the perimeter, i.e. the patient's face being tilted forward.

Dermatochalasis is a common upper lid disorder in which there is redundancy of the upper eyelid skin. It is often associated with protrusion of orbital fat through weakened orbital septum. Kosmin *et al.* (1997) studied 15 abnormal visual fields of nine ocular hypertensive eyes that appeared to have healthy optic discs. Dermatochalasis was found to be the underlying cause of supero-temporal quadrant field defects in the majority of cases (13/15). In seven cases, the superior field defect extended to the blind spot, mimicking a superior arcuate scotoma.

These problems have, again, been reported to have a higher incidence in automated as opposed to manual perimetry (Brenton *et al.*, 1986).

ACCURACY OF FIXATION

During an examination of the visual field it is of paramount importance that the patient maintains accurate fixation. If the patient does not then the results will show an increased variability. In kinetic

perimetry the isopter positions will keep changing and in threshold static perimetry there will be increased fluctuation.

While at the beginning of the examination the importance of accurate fixation can be emphasized to the patient, it is also important to have a means of monitoring fixation throughout the examination. If it is seen to vary then appropriate action can be taken, e.g. telling the patient to keep their eye still. The current generation of perimeters incorporate a variety of fixation monitoring devices.

Fixation monitoring by observation

The simplest technique for monitoring fixation is observation by the perimetrist. The observation can be direct, as is the case in most tangent screen instruments or with the aid of a telescope or camera, as is the case in most bowl perimeters. Such techniques are totally dependent upon the perimetrist's judgement and continued vigilance. The fact that the perimetrist needs to be present in order to make this judgement is an obvious disadvantage. As is the lack of any formal way for the perimetrist to comment on the accuracy of fixation.

The technique has been shown to have a good correlation with precise measures of fixation, which

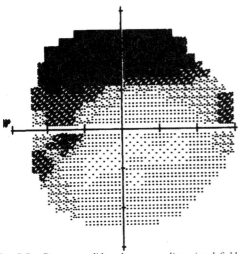
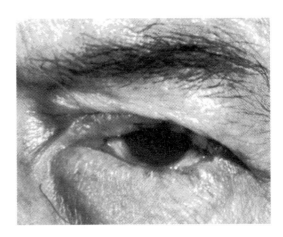

Fig. 5.5 *Droopy eyelid and corresponding visual field defect.*

is more than can be said for some of the more sophisticated techniques.

Automatic monitoring of fixation

The perimeter itself can incorporate a fixation monitor that either indicates to the perimetrist when fixation is inaccurate or, in the more sophisticated instruments, automatically repeats any measurements made while fixation was inaccurate. This is a very attractive option as it is both totally objective and does not require the perimetrist to be continually vigilant. However, like all good ideas, there is a problem. Most fixation monitors cannot differentiate between rotations of the eye, which occur when the patient looks away from the fixation target, and translations of the eye, which occur when the patient fidgets (a not uncommon event) (see Figure 5.6). A translation of the eye, such as a slight sideways movement of the head, does not necessarily mean that fixation has been lost or that the angular subtence of the perimetric stimuli has been changed by a large amount. A 10 mm lateral displacement of the eye will only change the angular subtence of a stimulus at 30 degrees by 1.7 degrees (Henson and Earlam, 1995).

In addition to the problems associated with differentiating between rotation and translation, automatic fixation monitors are generally insensitive to small, but significant, fixation errors (e.g. 1 degree). Some of the early computerized perimeters had automatic fixation monitors whose sensitivity could be varied.

It was soon evident, to anybody who used these instruments, that if the fixation monitor was set to be sensitive to small fixation inaccuracies (≤ 3 degree) then the incidence of fixation errors became so great that it was almost impossible to record any data. The solution was to either turn the fixation monitor off or to lower its sensitivity. While the latter approach may have given perimetrists a sense of well-being, in that they believed fixation was being monitored, in reality it was so crude as to be practically worthless.

Now you may be asking yourself, why do they not incorporate more accurate fixation monitors that are not fooled by translation effects? Well the answer is that there is no simple, easy-to-use reliable fixation monitor that can do this. In the research laboratory we can differentiate between rotations and translations by looking at the relative positions of the first and forth Purkinje images. The problem is that you need a clear lens, a large pupil and a stack of computer hardware. The first two requirements are surprisingly rare in the typical population of patients scheduled for perimetry.

Heijl–Krakau technique for sampling fixation

With this technique stimuli are occasionally presented in the region of the patient's blind spot. If fixation is accurate during these presentations the stimulus will not be seen. If, on the other hand, fixation is inaccurate then the stimulus is likely to fall outside of the blind spot and elicit a response. The results of this technique

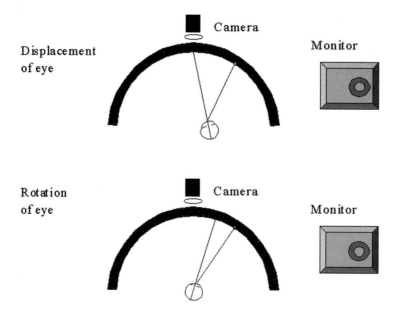

Fig. 5.6   *The difference between a displacement of the eye (top) with accurate fixation and rotation of the eye (bottom) with loss of fixation.*

are usually presented in the form of a fraction in which the numerator represents the number of times the patient reported seeing the blind spot stimulus and the denominator gives the number of times it was presented.

A frequently quoted fixation criteria for accepting the results of a visual field test is if the number of fixation errors is <33%. There is no evidence on which to base this cut-off value and the relatively small number of fixation tests (on average there are only 10–12 fixation tests in a perimetric test) mean that the precision of the estimated percentage is very low.

As the position of the blind spot varies from one individual to another it is necessary, at the onset of the examination to have a little routine which establishes the blind spot's location. The accuracy of this routine is important as errors may later manifest themselves as numerous fixation errors in a patient who has maintained good fixation. In a study which utilized an accurate eye position monitor during perimetric testing (Henson *et al.*, 1996) there was a poor correlation between the reported accuracy of fixation using the Heijl–Krakau technique and true error. The perimetrist opinion, derived from watching the patient's eye on a fixation monitor, was found to be better.

Figure 5.7 shows an optic nerve head upon which has been superimposed the standard Goldmann size III target (angle of subtence ≈0.5 degrees). As can be seen from the figure, the target is quite small in comparison to the optic disc. The patient's fixation is going to have to be quite a long way out for the stimulus to fall outside of the blind spot. In other words, this technique is not going to be very sensitive to small fixation errors.

The major advantages of the Heijl–Krakau technique are its simplicity and ease of implementation. Its disadvantages are:

1. It only samples fixation. Ideally, fixation should be monitored every time a stimulus is presented.
2. It increases the examination time.
3. It is unlikely to detect small fixation errors.

So what can we conclude about fixation monitors? It appears that, at present, the best fixation monitor is the perimetrist looking at an image of the eye displayed on a monitor. This technique is not only sensitive but, via verbal feedback, can result in an improvement in the fixation accuracy for subsequent presentations. It is helpful if the perimetrist's judgement is backed up by an objective estimate derived from a technique such as that proposed by Heijl and Krakau.

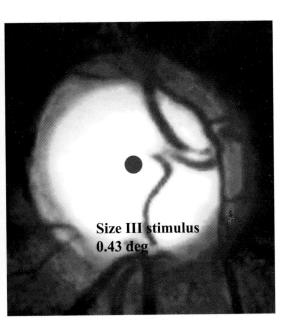

Fig. 5.7 *Size III stimulus superimposed upon an image of the optic nerve head.*

Perimetrists should, however, be encouraged to write on the record chart when they believe that the 'automatic' system has given an erroneous impression of the patient's fixation accuracy.

FIXATION TARGETS
During a visual field examination the patient is asked to fixate a continuously visible target which is attached to the perimeter. The size of this target is important. It needs to be small enough to encourage accurate fixation and big enough to be easily seen. It is common to have a separate target for patients with macular scotoma. This is often a large cross or four peripheral points, the patient being asked to fixate its perceived centre. Patients with macular scotoma can easily perceive where the centre of the pattern is and fixate with reasonable accuracy (Henson *et al.* 1998).

Also important is the contrast of the target. It needs to have high contrast elements to ensure an accurate accommodative response in those patients who still have some accommodation. If the patient does not accommodate accurately then the target will be blurred producing an effect similar to defocus (see p. 53).

Finally, it is important that the target is not too bright with respect to its background as this can cause local adaptation effects, which will lower the sensitivity of the neighbouring regions of the retina.

PROVISION OF AN AUDIBLE TONE PRIOR TO STIMULUS PRESENTATION
Many perimeters have the option of presenting an audible tone approximately 0.5 seconds before the stimulus/i are presented. This audible tone is designed to catch the patient's attention and prepare the patient for the visual stimulus.

The logic behind the provision of this facility is that the better prepared and more attentive the patient is the more reliable will be the results. To my knowledge there is no evidence to support this conclusion within the perimetric literature, although within the discipline of psychophysics there is considerable evidence to show that the provision of such stimuli will significantly improve the results.

PATIENT EXPERIENCE – THE LEARNING EFFECT
It has been known for some time that performance in a visual field examination improves as the patient gains experience with the test. This effect, which results in an apparent increase in the patient's sensitivity and a reduction in the amount of variability, is known as a learning effect.

The effect of learning, on static full-threshold techniques, has been investigated in both 'normal' and glaucomatous patients.

Wood *et al.* (1987a) found that normal subjects could be divided into three categories:

1. Those that show a gradual increase in their sensitivity across the five sessions analysed.
2. Those in whom no obvious improvement in sensitivity could be found.
3. Those in whom there was a large increase in sensitivity from the first to the second session which levels off on subsequent sessions.

They also noted that the increase in sensitivity was not consistent across the whole visual field, it often being greater in the superior compared to the inferior field and in the periphery as compared to the central field. Wood *et al.* (1987a) hypothesized that the larger increase in the superior field may be due to their subjects learning to raise their upper eyelid during the examination. The effect of eccentricity, which has also been noted by Heijl *et al.* (1989), has been ascribed to the concept that the peripheral field is a relatively unpractised sensory area.

The effect on glaucomatous eyes is similar to that found in normals (Wild *et al.*, 1989). The mean sensitivity increases with experience while the variability in results, as measured by the short-term fluctuation index, decreases. In the majority of cases the learning effect is fairly rapid, levelling off after the first examination of the first eye. In this situation the second eye will show very little learning effect in comparison to the first.

The existence of a learning effect, the amplitude of which can vary from one individual to another, has led several research groups to suggest that the first (Flammer *et al.*, 1984) or first two sessions (Wilensky and Joorndeph, 1984) should be ignored. The results of Wood *et al.* (1987a) suggest that the learning effect is, in the majority of case, fairly rapid and largely complete after the first examination of the first eye. In this situation it would only be necessary to repeat the examination of the first eye.

The effect of learning on kinetic perimetry has not been systematically evaluated. It would be expected that the position of the isopters would extend more towards the peripheral field and the variability would decrease as the patient gains experience with the test. It can also be expected that the learning effect would be greater with the more peripheral isopters. Kinetic perimetry is, however, subject to more operator bias than the static techniques described above. Skilled perimetrists will often repeat some of the first measurements, thereby reducing the effects of learning on the final field chart.

FATIGUE EFFECTS

Patient fatigue manifests itself as either an increase in the threshold or an increase in fluctuation. These effects are not due to an actual fatiguing of the visual system but rather to difficulties in the maintenance of attention.

In patients exerting accommodative effort during a visual field examination, fatigue may manifest itself as an inability to sustain this effort thereby producing effects similar to defocus.

Fatigue in normal patients

In normal patients the effects are minimal, being in the order of 1–1.5 dB when the threshold is measured continuously over a period of 30 minutes (Heijl, 1977; Heijl and Drance 1985), although Rabineau *et al.* (1985) reported a smaller increase in sensitivity when subjects were examined continuously for approximately 1 hour.

Fatigue in glaucoma patients

What is particularly interesting is that glaucoma patients show an enhanced fatigue-like effect, the overall magnitude of which is dependent upon whether the test location is in:

1. A relatively normal region of the field, in which case the effect is minimal and similar to that seen in normal patients.
2. A defective region of the field, in which case the fatigue effects are much larger having an average extent of nearly 6 dB (Heijl and Drance, 1985).
3. An area adjacent to a defective region of the field, in which case there is an increased fatigue effect similar in magnitude to that found in defective regions.

It is important to note that damaged locations of the visual field also show an enhanced variability in their responses (see Chapter 7).

Fatigue and examination strategy

Fatigue effects are also dependent upon the examination strategy. Fully automated techniques place considerable demands upon the patient with respect to maintaining their attention. Semi-automated techniques, in which the patient is given verbal feedback during the examination, help to maintain attention and reduce the effects of fatigue (De Jong *et al.*, 1985; Henson and Anderson, 1989). Threshold strategies are also found to be more demanding/fatiguing than suprathreshold strategies.

Reducing fatigue effects

Verbal encouragement helps to reduce fatigue effects as will interruption of the test sequence with rest periods.

LENS AND MEDIA OPACITIES

Lens and media opacities have two effects upon retinal sensitivity:

1. They act as a filter, reducing the amount of light reaching the retina.
2. They scatter the incoming light, reducing the contrast of any stimuli.

Since the filtering effect of media opacities will reduce the intensity of both the stimulus and the background, the contrast (ratio of the stimulus intensity to the background intensity) remains constant. Its effect will, due to the Weber–Fechner law, be less than expected on the basis of transmission (Heuer *et al.*, 1987) (see p. 52, Pupil effects).

The scattering effect of any opacity will, however, reduce the sensitivity since it affects the contrast of the stimuli. In a study by Guthauser *et al.* (1987) a correlation was found between the amount of back-scattered light from cataractous lenses and the attenuation of sensitivity. Similar results have been obtained from investigations in which scattering is induced in normal eyes (Heuer *et al.*, 1989; Urner-Bloch, 1987; Wood *et al.*, 1987b). While a correlation between back-scattered light and attenuation of sensitivity has been established it should be remembered that it is the forward-scattering of light that influences the threshold and that the above relationship with back-scattered light is merely a reflection of a relationship between forward- and back-scattered light.

When monitoring patients over a period of time it is important to know the likely effects of a cataract on the visual field and what will happen if the cataract is removed. A number of papers have investigated the effects of cataract removal (see Smith *et al.*, 1997; Chen and Budenz 1998). They have found that there is an increase in the overall sensitivity (mean defect and mean deviation) which is dependent upon the extent of the cataract, the increase being more evident at the central part of the visual field. The increase is not large, being less than 2 dB in cases where there is an early to moderate cataract. Visual field indices designed to identify focal visual field loss (loss variance and pattern standard deviation) show little change when cataracts are removed.

The effect of corneal (Faschinger, 1987) and vitreous opacities will again depend upon the scattering and absorption properties of the disturbance.

APHAKIA

Aphakia, absence of the crystalline lens, is usually the result of cataract surgery. Removal of a cataract will obviously have a significant effect upon the clarity of the retinal image (see previous section). It may also, depending upon the type of refractive correction, increase the magnification of the retinal image.

There are three types of refractive correction given to aphakics and each will have a very different effect upon the retinal image size:

1. Intra-ocular lens implants. These have no significant effect upon the retinal image size.
2. Contact lenses. These increase the size of the retinal image by approximately 9%, a value that, as far as perimetry is concerned, is insignificant.
3. Spectacle lenses. These increase the image size by approximately 30% and, hence, have a significant effect upon the perimetric result. Such large increases will result in an apparent contraction of the charted visual field. The blind spot will appear smaller and closer to the fixation point, the isopters closer to fixation and the peripheral sensitivities reduced.

These effects are due, solely, to the fact that field charts represent eccentricity in terms of the angle subtended at the eye rather than in terms of retinal coordinates. After a patient has received a spectacle correction for aphakia (or indeed any refractive error) the same retinal location will appear at a different location on the field chart. The magnitude of the induced change is dependent upon a number of factors:

1. The position of the correcting lens. The closer the correction is to the original position of the crystalline lens, the less it will affect the magnification.
2. The power of the correcting lens. The more powerful the correcting lens, the greater will be its effect.

ANGIOSCOTOMA

The central retinal artery and vein pass out of the optic disc and then branch into a number of divisions that spread out over the internal surface of the retina. Because these vessels lie in front of the visual cells they can mask the receptors from a stimulus. It is, in fact, possible with small stimuli on a 2 m Bjerrum screen to plot the course of the retinal vessels, although for this to be successful the subject needs to have a very stable fixation.

With static techniques of investigation, angioscotoma show up as the occasional missed stimulus, which, because of the size and location of these vessels, is more likely to occur near the blind spot and along the superior and inferior arcades (Henson *et al.*, 1984). The effects are also more likely to show up with small rather than large stimuli.

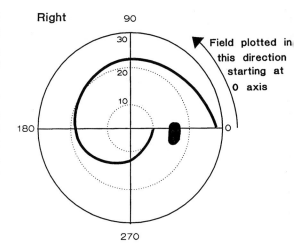

Fig. 5.8   *Result from hysteric patient.*

FUNCTIONAL FIELD LOSS (MALINGERING AND HYSTERIA)

The term functional loss is used to suggest that the impairment is a matter of function rather than structure (Thompson, 1985). This means that the retina, optic nerve and visual pathways are not physically damaged.

Patients with functional loss vary from the deliberate malingerer, who feigns visual loss, to the highly suggestive hysteric.

Visual field defects associated with the malingering patient are typically a contraction of the field with steep gradients at the edge. The malingerer can often be exposed by altering the testing distance and checking that the diameter of the defects adjusts itself according to the laws of physics, i.e. as the patient moves away from the screen the defect should cover a larger area.

The same type of defect is often found in the hysteric patient, and again altering the testing distance can often expose it. A second type of defect associated with hysteria is the spiral field (see Figure 5.8). This occurs in kinetic perimetry when the patient's hysteria produces a smaller and smaller field as the examination progresses. It is, of course, dependent upon the perimetrist plotting the field in a regular clockwise or anticlockwise manner. When the second eye is tested, or the first eye repeated, the patient normally exhibits a severely constricted tubular field.

An important aspect of the hysteric field is the susceptibility of the patient to suggestions. The extent and nature of field loss is thus dependent upon the perimetrist (Weller and Wiedemann, 1989).

When functional disorders are investigated with automated static perimetry, where there is no regular sequence of presentations, it is very difficult to differentiate them from genuine organic loss (Smith and Baker, 1987). Reliability indices are not helpful, false positives are uncommon, false negatives, where the patient fails to respond to an already seen stimulus, are often elevated but not out of proportion to that seen in severe organic loss. Fixation losses, as measured by blind spot presentations, are again within normal limits.

ADAPTATION

When someone passes from a light environment to a dark one it takes the eyes a few moments to adjust. This process is known as dark adaptation. If a visual field examination is started before the eyes have adapted to the background level then the first few sets of results will tend to be inaccurate.

The time needed for the eye's sensitivity to stabilize depends upon both the background intensity of the instrument being used and the prior level of adaptation. The greater the difference the longer it will take for the eye to stabilize. Most visual field instruments have background intensities that are in the upper mesopic/lower photopic range. Adaptation to these levels, from normal room illumination levels, takes only a few moments and is often complete by the time the patient has been instructed as to the nature of the test and run through a demonstration. To help this process along it is advisable to reduce the illumination before giving instructions, as this will give more time for the eyes to adapt.

A problem can arise when the patient's fundus has been examined prior to the visual field examination. The intensity of the light source used in examining the fundus is so high that it can take several minutes for the patient's threshold to return to normal. It is, therefore, not advisable to perform a visual field examination immediately after a fundus examination.

CONCLUSIONS

At the onset of this chapter I mentioned how frustrating it was to find, at the end of an examination, you had forgotten to include a refractive correction or omitted to tell the patient to keep their eyes wide open. I then asked whether in such situations it was really necessary to repeat the examination or whether the omission could be compensated for without jeopardizing its value.

In general the answer to this question is yes, providing certain preconditions are met. However, before going onto describe these preconditions it is important to question whether or not the omission can be corrected for by simply repeating a few of the measurements. For example, in the case of a lens rim artefact it would be better to simply re-test the defect areas with the correcting lens removed and then correct the chart accordingly. Unfortunately, this simple remedy can only be applied with a few perimeters. Most do not permit re-testing of a few locations followed by the printing out of a corrected field chart.

The preconditions that should apply before accepting the results of an examination known to incorporate artefacts are:

(a) any localized defects should be in an area of the visual field which is (i) recognized as being frequently affected by the uncorrected parameter and (ii) unlikely to be involved in any suspect pathology;

(b) any generalized depression should be relatively constant across the whole measured field.

This chapter has highlighted many of the problems that can occur during visual field measurement. Awareness of these problems is the secret of good perimetry. Once the perimetrist knows what can go wrong, then it is invariably quite simple to ensure that it does not.

REFERENCES

Atchison D.A. (1987) Effect of defocus on visual field measurement. *Ophthal Physiol Optics*, 7, 259–265.

Baldwin L.B. and Smith T.J. (1987) Does higher background illumination lessen the effect of media opacities on visual fields. *Doc Ophthalmol Proc Series*, 49, 65–68.

Benedetto M.D. and Cyrlin M.N. (1985) The effect of blur upon static perimetric thresholds. *Doc Ophthalmol Proc Series*, 42, 563–567.

Brenton R.S. and Phelps C.D. (1986) The normal visual field on the Humphrey Visual Field Analyzer. *Ophthalmologica*, 193, 56–74.

Brenton R.S., Phelps C.D., Rojas P. and Woolson R.F. (1986) Interocular differences of the visual field in normal subjects. *Invest Ophthalmol*, 27, 799–805.

Chen P.P. and Budenz D.L. (1998) The effect of cataract on the visual field of eyes with chronic open-angle glaucoma. *Am J Ophthalmol*, 125, 325–333.

Davson H. (1972) *The Physiology of the Eye*, 3rd edn. Churchill Livingstone, London.

De Jong D.G.M.M., Greve E.L., Bakker D. and Van Den Berg T.J.T.P. (1985) Psychological factors in computer assisted perimetry; automatic and semiautomatic perimetry. *Doc Ophthalmol Proc Series*, 42, 137–146.

Drance S.M., Berry V. and Hughes A. (1967) The effect of age on the central isopter of the normal visual field. *Can J Ophthalmol*, 2, 79–82.

Edgar D.F., Crabb D.P., Rudnicka A.R., Lawrenson J.G., Guttridge N.M. and O Brien C.J. (1999) Effects of dipivefrin and pilocarpine on pupil diameter, automated perimetry and LogMAR acuity. *Arch Ophthalmol*, 237, 117–124.

Faschinger C. (1987) Computer perimetry in patients with corneal dystrophies. *Doc Ophthalmol Proc Series*, 49, 61–64.

Flammer J., Drance S.M. and Zulauf M. (1984) Differential light threshold. Short and long term fluctuations in patients with glaucoma, normal controls and patients with suspected glaucoma. *Arch Ophthalmol*, 102, 876–879.

Guthauser U., Flammer J. and Niesel P. (1987) Relationship between cataract density and visual field damage. *Doc Ophthalmol Proc Series*, 49, 39–41.

Haas A., Flammer J. and Schneider U. (1986) Influence of age on the visual fields of normal subjects. *Am J Ophthalmol*, 101, 199–203.

Hart W.M. and Becker B. (1977) Visual field changes in ocular hypertension: computer-based analysis. *Arch Ophthalmol*, 95, 1176–1179.

Heijl A. (1977) Time changes of contrast thresholds during automatic perimetry. *Acta Ophthalmol*, 55, 696–708.

Heijl A. and Drance S.M. (1985) Deterioration of thresholds in glaucoma patients during perimetry. *Doc Ophthalmol Proc Series*, 42, 129–136.

Heijl A., Lindgren E. and Olsson J. (1987) Normal variability of static perimetric threshold values across the central visual field. *Arch Ophthalmol*, **105**, 1544–1549.

Heijl A., Lindgren E. and Olsson J. (1989) The effect of perimetric experience in normal subjects. *Arch Ophthalmol*, **107**, 81–86.

Henson D.B. and Anderson R. (1989) Thresholds using single and multiple stimulus presentations. In *Perimetry Update 1988/89* (ed. Heijl A.). Kugler & Ghedini, Amsterdam.

Henson D.B., Artes P.H. and Joseph A. (1998) Fixation errors during perimetry with central and peripheral fixation targets. *Invest Ophthalmol Vis Sci*, **39**, S24.

Henson D.B., Dix S. and Oborne A.C. (1984) Evaluation of the Friedmann Visual Field Analyser Mark II. Part 1. Results from a normal population. *Br J Ophthalmol*, **68**, 458–462.

Henson D.B. and Earlam R.A. (1995) Correcting lens system for perimetry. *Ophthalmic Physiol Opt*, **15**, 59–62.

Henson D.B., Evans J., Chauhan B.C. and Lane C. (1996) Influence of fixation accuracy on threshold variability in patients with open angle glaucoma. *Invest Ophthalmol Vis Sci*, **37**, 444–450.

Henson D.B. and Morris E.J. (1993) Effect of uncorrected refractive errors upon central visual field testing. *Ophthalmic Physiol Opt*, **13**, 339–343.

Heuer D.K., Anderson D.R., Feuer W.J. and Gressel M.G. (1989) The influence of decreased retinal illumination on automated perimetric threshold measurements. *Am J Ophthalmol*, **108**, 643–650.

Jaffe G.J., Alvarado J.A. and Juster R.P. (1986) Age-related changes of the normal visual field. *Arch Ophthalmol*, **104**, 1021–1025.

Johnson C.A., Adams A.J. and Lewis R.A. (1989) Evidence for a neural basis of age-related visual field loss in normal observers. *Invest Ophthalmol*, **30**, 2056–2064.

Johnson C.A. and Choy D. (1987) On the definition of area-related norms for visual function testing. *Applied Optics* **26**, 1449–1454.

Kosmin A.S., Wishart P.K. and Birch M.K. (1997) Apparent glaucomatous visual field defects caused by dermatochalasis. *Eye* **11**, 682–686.

Lindenmuth K.A., Skuta G.L., Rabbani R. and Musch D.C. (1989) Effect of pupillary constriction on automated perimetry in normal eyes. *Ophthalmol*, **96**, 1289–1301.

Mikelberg F.S., Drance S.M., Schultzer M. and Wijsman K. (1987) The effects of miosis on visual field indices. *Doc Ophthalmol Proc Series*, **49**, 645–649.

Millodot M. (1981) Effect of ametropia on peripheral refraction. *Am J Optom Physiol Optics*, **51**, 691–695.

Millodot M. and Millodot S. (1988) Presbyopia correction and the accommodation in reserve. *Ophthalmic Physiol Opt*, **9**, 126–132.

Rabineau P.A., Gloor B.P. and Tobler H.J. (1985) Fluctuations in threshold and effect of fatigue in automated static perimetry. *Doc Ophthalmol Proc Series*, **42**, 25–33.

Sloan L.L. (1960) Area and luminance of test object a variables in examination of visual field by projection perimetry. *Vis Res*, **1**, 121–138.

Smith T.J. and Baker R.S. (1987) Perimetric findings in functional disorders using automated techniques. *Ophthalmol*, **94**, 1562–1566.

Smith S.D., Katz J. and Quigley H.A. (1997) Effect of cataract extraction on the results of automated perimetry in glaucoma. *Arch Ophthalmol*, **115**, 1515–1519.

Thompson H.S. (1985) Functional visual loss. *Am J Ophthalmol*, **100**, 209–213.

Urner-Bloch U. (1987) Simulation of the influence of lens opacities on the perimetric results; investigated with orthoptic occluders. *Doc Ophthalmol Proc Series*, **49**, 23–31.

Webster A.R., Luff A.J., Canning C.R. and Elkington A.R. (1993) The effect of pilocarpine on the glaucomatous visual field. *Br J Ophthalmol*, **77**, 721–725.

Weinreb R.N. and Perlman J.P. (1986) The effect of refractive correction on automated perimetric thresholds. *Am J Ophthalmol*, **101**, 706–709.

Weller M. and Wiedemann P. (1989) Hysterical symptoms in ophthalmology. *Doc Ophthalmol*, **73**, 1–33.

Werner E.B., Adelson A. and Krupin T. (1988) Effect of patient experience on the results of automated perimetry in clinically stable glaucoma patients. *Ophthalmol*, **95**, 764–767.

Wild J.M., Dengler-Harles M., Searle A.E.T., O'Neill E.C. and Crews S.J. (1989) The influence of the learning effect on automated perimetry in patients with suspected glaucoma. *Acta Ophthalmol*, **67**, 537–545.

Wilensky J.T. and Joondeph B.C. (1984) Variations in visual field measurements with an automated perimeter. *Am J Ophthalmol*, **97**, 328–331.

Williams T.D. (1983) Aging and central visual field area. *Am J Optom Physiol Optics*, **60**, 888–891.

Wood J.M., Wild J.M., Bullimore M.A.and Gilmartin B. (1988) Factors affecting the normal perimetric profile derived by automated static threshold LED perimetry. I. Pupil size. *Ophthalmic Physiol Opt*, **8**, 26–31.

Wood J.M., Wild J.M., Hussey M.K. and Crews S.J. (1987a) Serial examination of the normal visual field using Octopus automated projection perimetry evidence for a learning effect. *Acta Ophthalmol*, **65**, 326–333.

Wood J.M., Wild J.M., Smerdon D.L. and Crews S.J. (1987b) The role of intraocular light scatter in the attenuation of perimetric response. *Doc Ophthalmol Proc Series*, **49**, 51–59.

Zalta A.H. (1989) Lens rim artefact in automated threshold perimetry. *Ophthalmol*, **96**, 1302–1311.

6 Visual pathways

INTRODUCTION

The course taken by the visual fibres from the retina through to the visual cortex is known as the primary visual pathway. While, as the name implies, the main function of the pathways is to transmit visual information from the eye to the cortex, it is important to realize that in doing so the fibres undergo a considerable amount of sorting and realignment while the visual signals also undergo a certain amount of processing in both the retina and the lateral geniculate body.

This chapter will deal with the primary visual pathway in the conventional manner, starting at the retina and then gradually proceeding through to the visual cortex. At each stage it will discuss:

(a) The relevant anatomical details.
(b) The common pathologies.
(c) The visual field defects which arise from these pathologies.

Inevitably, this chapter will include a weighty amount of material for the reader to digest and in an attempt to make this information more 'digestible', and to help the clinician who is left looking at a visual field chart wondering what the result really means, a series of flow charts have been included at the end of this chapter to help those intent on making a diagnosis on the basis of visual field data.

Before getting immersed in the details of the visual pathways there are two features of visual field defects that it would be well to discuss now: these are congruity and macular sparing.

Congruity

I have already briefly mentioned that the fibres

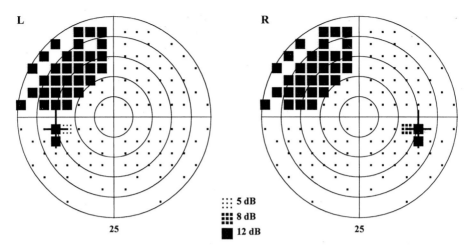

Fig. 6.1 *Congruous field defect. With the exception of the locations representing the optic disc, in the temporal region of each field chart, the visual field defects are exactly the same in both eyes.*

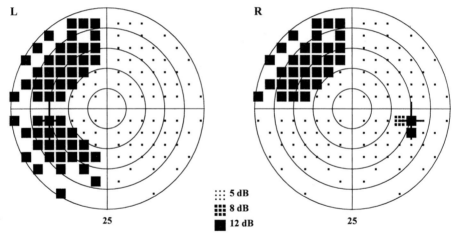

Fig. 6.2 *Incongruous field defect. The field defect in the right eye is larger, extending to the inferior visual field, than that of the left eye.*

undergo a considerable amount of sorting and alignment as they travel from the retina to the visual cortex. Indeed, during this passage, the nerves that represent corresponding points in the two eyes (points which view the same object) get closer and closer together. Lesions of the visual cortex, therefore, often produce perfectly congruous (identical in both eyes) visual field defects (see Figure 6.1), while those from the optic tracts often produce incongruous defects (see Figure 6.2). This characteristic can be valuable in localizing the position of a lesion.

Of course congruity only applies to the binocular part of the visual field. Perimetrists must be careful not to label field defects as incongruous simple because they extend into a monocular region of the visual field.

Macular sparing

Macular sparing is when the central 5–10 degrees of the visual field is unaffected in an otherwise hemianopic defect (a defect that affects one half of the field). It is a common characteristic of visual field defects arising from supra-geniculate lesions (see Figure 6.3).

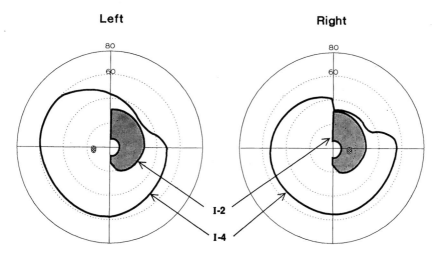

Fig. 6.3 *Macular sparing. The hemianopic defect, affecting the right visual field, does not include the macular region.*

Numerous explanations have been put forward to account for macular sparing, many of which have now been refuted as new evidence has come to light (see Ehlers, 1975 for a review of these). Currently, there are three plausible theories:

(1) Shifts in ocular fixation.
(2) Separate blood supply.
(3) Extent of macular representation.

Shifts in ocular fixation

Patients with hemianopic defects may learn to view objects of interest eccentrically in order to ensure that half of it is not lost within the field defect. In fact, such techniques are regularly taught to partially sighted patients with macular lesions. The theory goes that these patients, when asked to look at the fixation target of the perimeter, continue to view slightly to one side, which results in an apparent macular sparing. Some recent work using a fundus perimeter – an instrument that allows the operator to view the fundus during perimetry and to locate the stimuli at a given retinal site – has demonstrated macular sparing in patients who do not show a shift in fixation (Rohrschneider *et al.*, 1997). This theory cannot, therefore, explain all cases of macular sparing.

Separate blood supply

The separate blood supplies theory follows from some work done by Smith and Richardson (1966). They demonstrated two interesting points: (i) in some individuals the occipital pole of the visual cortex is supplied by the middle cerebral artery rather than the posterior cerebral artery and (ii) in some patients, there is a horizontal border at the macular between the areas supplied by the posterior temporal artery (a branch of the posterior cerebral artery) and the area supplied by the middle cerebral artery.

Both these findings could explain macular sparing. If an occlusion occurs in either the posterior cerebral artery in a patient whose macular area is supplied by the middle cerebral artery, or in a branch of the posterior cerebral artery which does not supply the macular area, then some macular sparing would result. Some clinical evidence supporting the latter explanation has been provided by Ehlers (1975), who reported on eight cases in which the macular sparing was confined to either the upper or lower quadrant.

The separate blood supply theory must not be confused with an earlier theory based upon the belief that there is a dual blood supply to the visual cortex. There is no anatomic evidence of a dual blood supply to the visual cortex (Glaser, 1978).

Extent of macular representation

The final theory to explain macular sparing simply states that the macular area has such a large cortical representation that in any incomplete lesion there is a high probability that some of the macular fibres will be left intact.

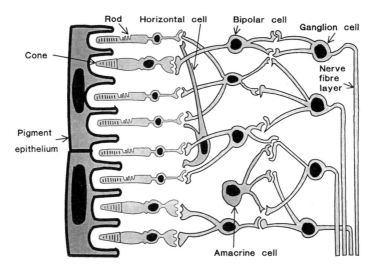

Fig. 6.4 *Schematic diagram of neural elements within the retina.*

Important caveat

Before leaving the introduction and delving into the different sections of the visual pathways there is another important caveat for all would-be perimetrists. There is always a tendency in texts such as this to try to categorize and, to some extent, simplify things in order to help understanding. An unfortunate side effect of this is that certain types of pathology become rigidly associated with certain types of field defect. A quick glance through the clinical journals will highlight the dangers of rigid association; there are many examples of atypical defects, which in some instances defy explanation even when the full details of the pathology are known. The student should always bear these in mind, remembering Murphy's law: if something can be atypical it almost always is!

RETINA

Anatomy

The retina contains two types of receptors, the rods and cones, which are responsible for converting light energy into a neural response. This response is transmitted to the bipolar cells and then onto the ganglion cells whose axons leave the eye via the optic nerve. The horizontal and amacrine cells connect laterally and act to modulate the visual response (see Figure 6.4).

The human retina contains some 120 million rods and 6 million cones whose density (number per solid angle) varies with retinal location. The cone density is greatest at the fovea, falling off abruptly, at an eccentricity of 10 degrees, to a relatively low level that then remains fairly constant across the remaining retina. The density of rods peaks at an eccentricity of 20 degrees, falling off to almost 0 at the fovea and to an intermediate level at eccentricities beyond 20 degrees.

Of more functional significance, due to the close relationship between cortical representation and ganglion cell density, is the relationship that exists between the density of ganglion cells and eccentricity. This varies from approx. two ganglion cells per receptor at the fovea to several hundred receptors per ganglion cell in the periphery. In comparison to receptor cell densities there is a fairly simple relationship between the density of ganglion cells and eccentricity (Drasdo, 1989).

An important fact for the perimetrist to take on board is that the bundle of fibres supplying the macula, the maculo-papillary bundle, accounts for approximately one-third of all retinal fibres.

Of particular importance to perimetry is the path followed by the ganglion cell axons from their origin within the outer nuclear layer of the retina to the optic nerve head. These axons (fibres) sweep across the inner surface of the retina to the optic nerve head where they turn through 90 degrees and exit from the globe as the optic nerve. The ganglion cell fibres lie anterior to the receptors and undoubtedly cause a certain amount of scatter at the receptor layer. To

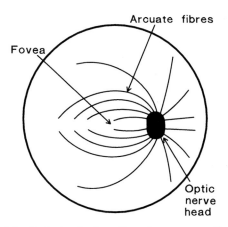

Fig. 6.5 *Retinal path of ganglion cell axons, nerve fibre layer. Note how they curve around the fovea and do not cross the horizontal midline.*

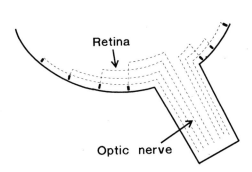

Fig. 6.6 *Retinal path of ganglion cell axons.*

avoid this scatter affecting the foveal region, where the eye's acuity reaches its highest level, the normal direct course of the ganglion cell fibres is altered. The fibres from the temporal side of the retina travel in arcs around the fovea (see Figure 6.5).

Ganglion cell fibres are also characterized by their failure to cross the horizontal midline. Any damage caused to these fibres, be it in the retina or at the optic nerve head, tends to respect this horizontal boundary. In contrast, defects that involve deeper layers of the retina do not respect this boundary. The horizontal midline, therefore, forms an important boundary for the recognition and localization of retinal pathology.

In addition to their characteristic course over the retina, ganglion cell fibres also have a vertical stratification. Axons from ganglion cells near the disc are more superficial than those that arise from the peripheral retina (see Figure 6.6).

The blood supply to the retina is divided into two parts. The outer retina is supplied from the choroidal vessels while the inner retina is supplied from the central retinal artery. This artery enters through the optic disc and, after dividing into four major branches, passes over the inner surface of the retina. Blood from the inner retina returns through the central retinal vein which exits through the optic nerve. The pattern of the retinal vessels is similar to that of the nerve fibres. They arc around the foveal region and do not cross the horizontal midline.

Visual field defects associated with retinal disorders

The optics of the eye both inverts and reverses the objects we look at, i.e. objects that we see in the superior field are imaged on the inferior retina and objects seen in the temporal field are imaged on the nasal retina. Any disorder of the retina, therefore, produces field defects in the opposite hemifield (see Table 6.1).

Lesions in the outer layers of the retina produce visual field defects that tend not to respect the vertical and horizontal midlines. In most cases there are observable ophthalmoscopic changes on which any diagnosis is largely based, e.g. age-related maculopathy, diabetic retinopathy. In such conditions visual field measures are helpful in assessing the extent of damage and occasionally in confirming a diagnosis.

It should be added, however, that the relationship between observable damage with the ophthalmoscope and visual field loss is often less than perfect. For example Hart and Burde (1983) reported that in 20% of patients with central scotoma resulting from macular disease there was a relative sparing at the point

Table 6.1 Relationship between retinal location and the visual field

Damage	Field defect
Inferior retina	Superior field
Nasal retina	Temporal field
Temporal retina	Nasal field
Superior retina	Inferior field

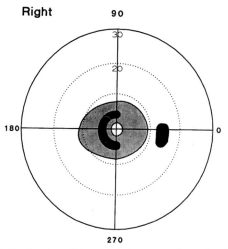

Right   **90**

Fig. 6.7 *Sparing of the macula in a case of macular disease.*

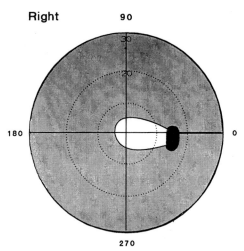

Right   **90**

Fig. 6.8 *Residual island of vision in case of central retinal artery occlusion with a cilioretinal artery.*

of fixation (see Figure 6.7). Such results would be difficult to predict from the ophthalmoscopic appearance. It is also interesting to note that Hart and Burde (1983) never found ring type defects in patients with optic nerve disease. This finding could, they feel, be of use in differential diagnosis.

Disorders of the inner retina, such as occlusions of the retinal vessels, produce defects which respect the horizontal midline and follow the course of the ganglion cell fibres; e.g. an occlusion of a branch of the retinal artery, see below.

Vascular occlusions

Occlusions of the central retinal artery cause an abrupt painless loss of vision and rapid death of the ganglion cells. In such cases the presence of a cilioretinal artery may lead to a residual island of vision usually in the central and centrocecal area (see Figure 6.8). Branch occlusions of the central retinal artery produce sector and arcuate defects, the exact location of the defect being dependent upon the affected branch (see Figure 6.9). Visual field defects associated with arterial occlusions are characterized by their permanence, and sharp edges.

Occlusions of the central retinal vein again cause an abrupt, painless loss of vision. In the majority of cases the acuity is reduced to less than 6/60 and there is little if any recovery even when followed for a number of years (Hill and Griffiths, 1970). Branch retinal vein occlusions give more variable results. While acuity is

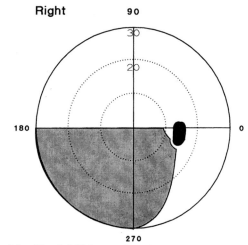

Right   **90**

Fig. 6.9 *Visual field loss resulting from a branch occlusion of the central retinal artery.*

often affected the loss is not as severe and the prognosis for recovery better (Hill and Griffiths, 1970). This is especially true in the younger patients where the extent of recovery is often surprising.

The haemorrhaging and oedema that follow a branch vein occlusion would be expected to produce irregular-shaped relative defects, which regress with the re-absorption of the blood. It is, however, not unusual to find cases where the defect is not only absolute and permanent but also follows the nerve fibre distribution. Investigation of these patients has demonstrated that, in addition to the vein occlusion, there is often some arterial disease and it is the arterial disease that has led to the more severe field loss (Birchall *et al.*, 1976).

Two important points to remember about venous occlusions are:

(1) they are common in patients with primary glaucoma; and
(2) they give rise to secondary glaucoma.

Nutritional and toxic optic neuropathies

Various nutritional deficiencies and certain drugs are known to produce retinal neuropathies. The effects are varied but primarily involve the central part of the visual field. This makes them particularly easy to detect with Amsler charts.

Vitamin deficiencies and tobacco-alcohol related amblyopia. The neuropathies related to nutritional deficiency and the abuse of tobacco and alcohol are normally grouped together because they present with identical clinical signs. Many clinicians believe that all three conditions are related, dietary deficiency being the common denominator. Prognosis for recovery is good although this can take a considerable time, 3–9 months. Treatment consists of a well-balanced diet with B-complex vitamin supplement.

Bilateral, relatively symmetrical, centrocecal scotoma (see Figure 6.10), are the most commonly reported type of field defect. The defects are most prominent with red or green targets, a manifestation of the acquired red/green dyschromatopsia that is often present in these patients. While field loss is often associated with reduced visual acuity, there have been reports of patients retaining normal acuity while having significant visual field loss and deficits in colour discrimination (Brusini *et al.*, 1987).

It is not known why these conditions have a predilection for the fibres supplying the centrocecal area or in fact why other types of toxic optic nerve neuropathies produce different types of field loss.

Chloroquine retinopathy. The antimalarial drugs, chloroquine phosphate and hydroxychloroquine sulphate, which are also used in the treatment of rheumatoid arthritis and other immunological diseases of connective tissue, are known to produce ocular damage in a (cumulative) dose-related fashion. Recent work has demonstrated that, in the case of hydroxychloroquine, it is not so much the cumulative dose that is associated with retinopathy but the size of the daily dose. Johnson and Vine (1987) found little evidence of any cumulative effect in patients taking daily doses of less than 400 mg/day. A particularly worrying aspect of this type of retinopathy is that once detected it often progresses even when the drug therapy is discontinued.

The types of ocular damage seen with chloroquine include corneal deposits, loss of accommodation and retinopathy, the latter being the most serious.

Visual field defects are central (within the central 30 degrees) and may or may not involve the macula. They can also be present when there are no observable ophthalmoscopic changes. The defects are more noticeable with red targets, although they can often

Left

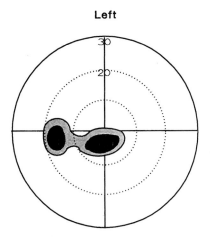

Right

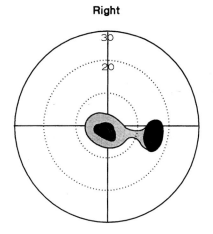

Fig. 6.10 *Centrocecal scotoma due to nutritional deficiency.*

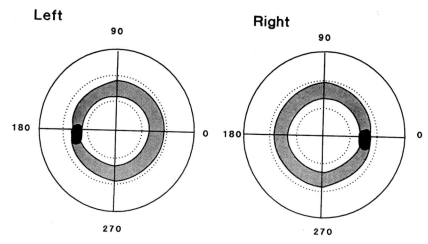

Fig. 6.11 *Perifoveal ring scotoma due to chloroquine retinopathy.*

be detected with white stimuli, especially when sensitive techniques, such as full-threshold perimetry, are used. One type of central field defect found in chloroquine retinopathy is a perifoveal ring depression (see Figure 6.11). This defect has been reported in a wide variety of macular pathologies, leading to the conclusion that it might be a stereotyped response of the retina to macular insults (Hart and Burde, 1983). It is the superior part of the central field that is often the most susceptible to damage.

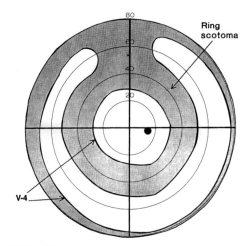

Fig. 6.12 *Ring scotoma in case of retinitis pigmentosa.*

Retinitis pigmentosa

Retinitis pigmentosa is a generic term used to describe a group of retinal degenerations. While it has for a long time been viewed as an inherited condition, with several different inheritance patterns, a significant number of cases appear to have no family history of the disorder (Boughman and Fishman, 1983).

The diagnosis of retinitis pigmentosa is based upon a number of factors, including:

- Night blindness.
- Progressive peripheral visual field loss.
- Bone spicule pigmentation in the mid-peripheral retina.
- Arterial attenuation.
- An attenuated or non-existent ERG.

There is no known treatment for retinitis pigmentosa and patients gradually, over a period of many years, lose more and more of their peripheral field until they

become totally blind or are left with only a small central island of vision. While loss of the central field does occur, either from the progressive nature of the degeneration or as a result of separate macular lesions, it is important to note that 25% of patients retain good central acuity throughout life.

Retinitis pigmentosa is associated with a variety of field defects which, in the early stages, are more pronounced when the background illumination is reduced. Loss of the peripheral field is an early sign, along with a ring scotoma, the outer edge of which is beyond the central 30 degrees (see Figure 6.12). The defects are bilaterally symmetrical and progress slowly until in the later stages there is either a complete loss of

Left **Right**

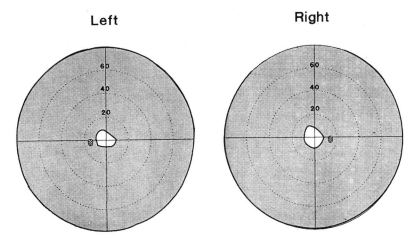

Fig. 6.13 *Advanced case of retinitis pigmentosa showing small residual central island of vision.*

vision or a small central island at the fovea (see Figure 6.13). While the rate of visual field loss was originally believed to be related to the mode of inheritance, more recent work has questioned this and suggested that it is the same in all genetic subtypes (Massof *et al.*, 1990).

Retinal detachments

Detachment of the retina normally occurs at the receptor/pigment epithelium border. The receptors are hence deprived of their blood supply and ultimately die.

Field defects are initially relative and correspond to the position and size of the detachment. In the case of simple detachments, the defects normally break through (extend out) to the periphery. In solid detachments, caused by neoplasms, the edge of the defect tends to be less severe and may not break through to the periphery.

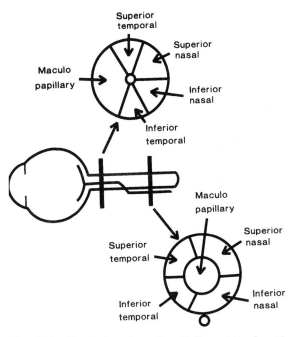

Fig. 6.14 *Distribution of ganglion cell fibres within the optic nerve.*

THE OPTIC NERVE

Anatomy

The optic nerve contains approximately 1 000 000 nerve fibres, each one arising from a single retinal ganglion cell. The optic nerve connects the eyeball to the optic chiasma and leaves the orbit via the optic canal. The distal portion, that part close to the eyeball, has the central retinal artery and vein running through its centre (see Figure 6.14).

When the ganglion cell axons enter the optic nerve they are distributed according to their retinal origin.

The axonal density is highest in the inferior temporal quadrant where the major portion of the papillomacular bundle enters the nerve.

As the ganglion cell axons progress down the nerve they redistribute themselves. The fibres from the peripheral parts of the retina eventually occupy the peripheral parts of the nerve and those from the central

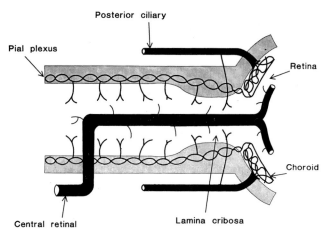

Fig. 6.15 *Blood supply to the optic nerve head.*

retina occupy the central part of the nerve (see Figure 6.14). Just behind the globe the axons receive myelin sheaths, which results in a considerable thickening of the nerve.

One particular region of the optic nerve that has received a great deal of attention by researchers, due to its association with glaucoma, is the optic nerve head. The blood supply to this region is particularly complex. While all of the blood supply originates from the ophthalmic artery, it arrives at the optic nerve head from three distinct vascular beds:

(a) The central retinal artery which passes down the centre of the optic nerve.
(b) The posterior ciliary arteries.
(c) The pial vasculature immediately behind the globe.

Figure 6.15 summarizes the contributions made by these three vascular beds. The blood supply is richly anastomotic although this may change with age or disease.

At the level of the lamina cribosa the axons are segregated into discrete bundles by interlaced connective tissue elements. Axons from adjacent ganglion cells are grouped together into fibre bundles and any lesions at this level would produce a localized visual field defect.

Visual field defects associated with optic nerve disorders
Glaucoma
One of the most common causes of damage to the optic

nerve head is glaucoma. The condition is of such importance to the perimetrist that a whole chapter has been devoted to it (see Chapter 7).

Tilted optic disc
A tilted optic disc is a congenital anomaly in which the optic disc appears tilted to the nasal rather than temporal side. It is also known as Fuchs coloboma, congenital crescents, conus, dysversion of the optic nerve head and situs inversus, the last name referring to the course of the emerging vessels, which tend to leave on the nasal rather than temporal side of the disc. It is bilateral in approximately 80% of cases.

Tilted optic disc is due to an abnormality at the optic nerve head that results in hypoplasia of the retina and choroid and ectasia of the fundus. It is associated with myopia and has a reported incidence of 3.41% (von Szily, 1922). The elevation of the disc margin has occasionally led to the suspicion of papilloedema.

The main type of visual field defect associated with tilted discs is a temporal depression which could easily be confused with chiasmal disorders, especially when the condition is bilateral (Graham and Wakefield, 1973; Young *et al.*, 1976; Brazitikos *et al.*, 1990) (see Figure 6.16). The depression does, however, often cross the vertical midline, a characteristic not found in chiasmal lesions. The defects are believed to be the result of diffuse hypoplasia of the optic nerve the inferior nasal sector of which is more affected. The defects are also more evident in the central field

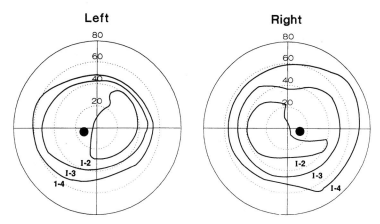

Fig. 6.16 *Field defect due to tilted optic disc. Note how the defect crosses the vertical midline.*

although they are not confined to it. The extent of visual field loss, as measured by the global index mean deviation, is positively related to the extent of myopia.

Drusen of the optic nerve head

Optic disc drusen are formed by the accumulation of deposits (chiefly calcified mitochondria) in the optic nerve head. It is a congenital defect that is thought to be related to the size of the lamina cribosa. The drusen tend to remain buried during the early years of life, becoming visible during the second and third decade when they appear as white swellings often extending beyond the disc margin. The incidence of optic disc drusen has been put at approximately 1% of the population although an investigation of cadaver eyes has suggested that it may be as high as 2% (Friedmann *et al.*, 1979). The condition is invariably bilateral and progressive although it rarely affects visual acuity. The best technique for identifying disc drusen is B-mode ultrasonography.

Visual field defects have been reported to occur in over 80% of cases (Lorentzen, 1966), and are generally relative and arcuate in nature (Gutteridge and Cockburn, 1981). The extent of visual field loss is dependent upon the size of the drusen which also cause a thinning of the nerve fibre layer (Roh *et al.*, 1998). The visual field defects are believed to result from the drusen pressing on the optic nerve bundles. There does not appear to be any correlation between the position of the drusen and the position of the field defect.

The field defects can be confused with those from glaucoma and the early ophthalmoscopic signs with papilloedema.

Anterior ischaemic optic neuropathy

Anterior ischaemic optic neuropathy results from acute ischaemia of the anterior part of the optic nerve (part supplied by the posterior ciliary artery). It is caused by circulatory occlusive disorders and is often associated with temporal arteritis and diabetes mellitus. It most often involves a segment of the nerve and only rarely involves the whole nerve.

Ophthalmic examination during the acute stage of this condition reveals optic disc oedema, the disc becoming atrophic usually within 2 months. Visual acuity is affected in the majority of cases, more so in those with temporal arteritis than those without. While some patients show a slight improvement with time to both their acuity and field loss, the majority are left with a severe disability. There is also a high incidence of the fellow eye becoming involved.

The type of field loss associated with anterior ischaemic optic neuropathy is dependent upon whether the temporal artery is involved (Hayreh and Podhajsky, 1979). In those with temporal arteritis the most significant finding is the extent of field loss. Hayreh and Podhajsky (1979) reported that 43% of their cases (168 eyes) had no recordable visual field and that a further 11% only had a peripheral island. The remainder of their group had a variety of central and peripheral defects. In cases where temporal arteritis was not present the most common form of

Left

Right

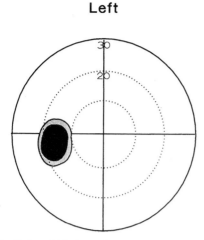
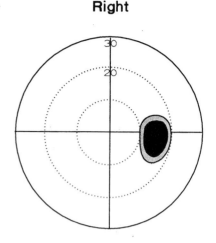

Fig. 6.17 *Enlarged blind spot due to papilloedema.*

defect was a central scotoma, inferior nasal and inferior altitudinal defects also being common.

Because the lesion in ischaemic optic neuropathy is sited at the optic nerve head, the visual field defects usually relate to the course of the retinal nerve fibres, often ending at the horizontal raphé. This means the defects can often resemble those seen in glaucoma (Aulhorn and Tanzil, 1979). Differences between the defects seen in anterior ischaemic optic neuropathy (AION) and glaucoma are:

(a) In AION the defects occur suddenly with the result that the patient is often aware of the visual field loss. Patients with primary open angle glaucoma are rarely aware of any field loss until is has reached a significant portion of their visual field.

(b) It is not uncommon for defects in AION to involve the inferior field and the macular. The macular, by comparison, is rarely involved in the early stages of glaucoma.

Despite these differences a differential diagnosis cannot be made solely on the basis of the visual field defects and must rely upon other factors such as ophthalmoscopic signs and intraocular pressure.

Papilloedema

Papilloedema, a non-inflammatory swelling of the disc, is caused by raised intra-cranial pressure. In early stages it is difficult to differentiate it from papillitis,

which is an inflammatory condition involving the optic nerve head (see following section for more details).

Papilloedema causes recognizable swelling at the nerve head. Patients have symptoms that relate to the raised intra-cranial pressure – headaches, diplopia and vomiting. The condition is bilateral and does not affect the visual acuity until it has reached an advanced stage.

The classic visual field defect found in papilloedema is bilaterally enlarged blind spots (see Figure 6.17), although this may not be present in the early stages. In later stages papilloedema can result in both peripheral and central loss. While release of the raised intra-cranial pressure can often result in a substantial recovery of the visual field, the amount of recovery is dependent upon the length of time and extent of the raised intra-cranial pressure. If the pressure has been raised for a significant amount of time then some optic atrophy will have occurred, resulting in permanent visual field loss.

Optic neuritis

Optic neuritis is a term used to describe a series of conditions that can affect both the optic nerve and nerve head. It includes both inflammations and demyelinating degenerations of the optic nerve. When it involves the nerve head, giving the ophthalmoscopic sign of a swollen disc, it is called papillitis. When it is confined to an area behind the disc, thereby giving no visible signs, it is called retrobulbar neuritis. Generally speaking papillitis is more common in children, while retrobulbar neuritis is more common in adults.

Optic neuritis can be classified according to whether it is:

- Idiopathic, no known cause.
- Due to demyelination.
- Miscellaneous, i.e. viral infections.

The visual symptoms associated with optic neuritis are:

- A rapid, progressive loss of central vision (usually reaches its lowest level after approximately 1 week).
- A tender globe, with pain on movement of eye.
- A normal fundus in the retrobulbar type and disc swelling in papillitis often with flame haemorrhages.

In the majority of cases, the vision returns in the second and third week and many patients enjoy normal or near normal return of acuity by the fourth or fifth week. Occasionally, however, the vision can take longer to improve or does not fully return.

Optic neuritis, particularly the retrobulbar type, is often associated with multiple sclerosis. Exact statistics on the subject vary enormously from one report to another. A recent review paper found that anywhere from 13 to 85% of patients who have an attack of optic neuritis have been reported to eventually develop multiple sclerosis and that 50% of patients with multiple sclerosis have electrophysiological and neuro-pathological evidence of previous optic neuritis (Sergott and Brown, 1988). The high incidence of electrophysiological and neuro-pathological evidence of optic neuritis may signify that in certain instances the attacks are sub-clinical and do not give rise to any symptoms. These patients may well have subtle visual field defects which do not involve the macula (which is one of the reasons why the patient does not report any symptoms) and which need sensitive techniques of investigation to detect.

Multiple sclerosis can also involve other regions of the visual pathways, such as the optic tracts and radiations. Manifest lesions of these tracts are, however, rare compared to those involving the optic nerve (Sanchez-Dalmau *et al.*, 1991).

Visual field loss in optic neuritis is invariably monocular, although it is feasible for both optic nerves to be involved. While several early papers refer to a predominance of centrocecal defects in optic neuritis, later work by Keltner *et al.* (1993) has shown a wide variety of defects, including diffuse loss, nerve fibre bundle defects and centrocecal loss.

The pattern of field loss reflects the region of nerve affected. If the central section is involved (axial neuritis) then there will be central field loss. If, on the other hand, only the peripheral section of the nerve is involved (periaxial neuritis) then the central field will be preserved.

The field defects associated with optic neuritis show a great deal of fluctuation and can change in both their size and extent from one day to the next. The existence of visual field loss during the symptomatic acute phase of optic neuritis is almost universal and common in asymptomatic eyes. The subtle nature of these defects, which are often relative (Meienberg *et al.*, 1985), led earlier reports to conclude that a number of patients with optic neuritis did not develop visual field defects.

Optic atrophy

Optic atrophy, which is a general term used to describe a degeneration of the optic nerve fibres and not a specific disease, can be evaluated and/or substantiated with visual field measures. Optic atrophy is characterized by a pallor of the optic nerve head that may appear greyish, yellowish or white. The wide range of normal disc appearances can make it difficult to establish whether the 'pallor' of a disc is physiological or pathological. If a visual field defect can be found, then this indicates that a pale disc is a true optic atrophy rather than physiological pallor. The nature of the field defect in optic atrophy is, of course, dependent upon its cause.

THE CHIASMA
Anatomy
The two optic nerves join together at the chiasma and the fibres from the nasal retinas cross over (decussate) before continuing on their journey, in what is now called the optic tracts, to the lateral geniculate body (see Figure 6.18).

It must be remembered that the nasal retina receives images from the temporal field and it is, therefore, the fibres from the temporal field which cross over in the chiasma. Thus, while each optic

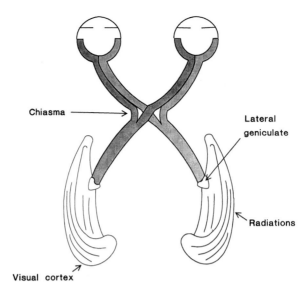

Chiasma

Lateral geniculate

Radiations

Visual cortex

Fig. 6.18 *Primary optic pathway.*

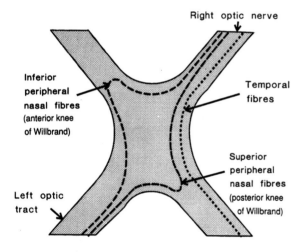

Right optic nerve

Inferior peripheral nasal fibres (anterior knee of Willbrand)

Temporal fibres

Superior peripheral nasal fibres (posterior knee of Willbrand)

Left optic tract

Fig. 6.19 *Course of fibres within the optic chiasma.*

nerve carries all the ganglion cell axons from one eye, each optic tract carries all the ganglion cell axons from either the right or left visual field. Axons from the right visual field are contained within the left optic tract and those from the left visual field in the right optic tract.

Because the temporal visual field is slightly larger than the nasal field, slightly more than 50% of the visual fibres decussate. Within the structure of the chiasma, the visual fibres are organized in a systematic manner (see Figure 6.19). The decussating fibres from the central part of the field cross in a broad band through the centre of the chiasma, those from the superior peripheral field cross in the anterior part while those from the inferior peripheral field cross in the posterior part. After crossing through the chiasma, the fibres from the superior peripheral field enter into the optic nerve of the opposite side for a short distance before doing a U-turn and passing into the optic tract. This kink into the optic nerve is known as the anterior knee of Willbrand and its presence has important clinical implications when it comes to localizing the site of any lesions. The fibres follow a similar, but not so pronounced, course from the inferior peripheral field. They pass into the optic tract for a short distance before doing their U-turn and then decussating to the optic tract on the opposite side. This kink is known as the posterior knee of Willbrand (see Figure 6.19).

Of particular interest to the perimetrist is the relationship of the chiasma to other anatomical structures and in particular its relationship to the pituitary gland (see Figure 6.20). Tumours of the pituitary gland can put pressure on the chiasma and cause characteristic patterns of visual field loss (see below for more details). The nature of any field loss is dependent upon many factors, one of which is the relative positions of the chiasma and pituitary gland. In the majority of patients the chiasma lies almost directly above the pituitary body while in approximately 16% of

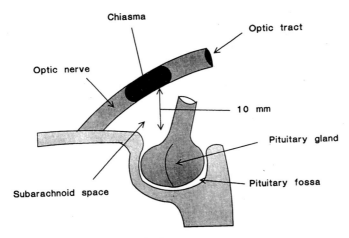

Fig. 6.20 *Relationship of chiasma to the pituitary gland.*

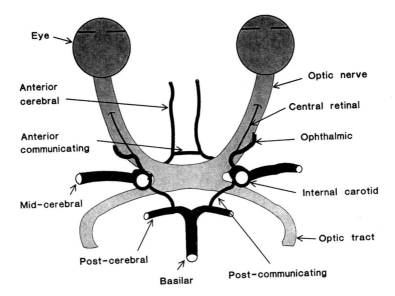

Fig. 6.21 *Relationship of chiasma to major cranial vessels.*

patients it lies anterior to the pituitary (a prefixed chiasma). In a further 4% it lies posterior to the pituitary (a post-fixed chiasma).

The chiasma is closely associated with a number of important blood vessels. On either side of it are the internal carotid arteries, in front and above are the anterior cerebral and communicating arteries and below and towards the optic tracts are the posterior cerebral and communicating arteries (see Figure 6.21). The arterial circle of Willis, which is made up of all the aforementioned arteries, actually surrounds the visual pathway at the optic chiasma.

Visual field defects associated with chiasmal disorders

The type of visual field loss resulting from lesions to the chiasma is dependent upon the site of the lesion. Figure 6.22 summarizes the many different types of field loss that can be expected from chiasmal lesions. While this figure gives a relatively clear and unambiguous description of the types of field loss associated with chiasmal lesions, it is not always possible to predict the site of the original lesion from the visual field defect. Other factors such as the nature of any tumour, be it hard or soft, its speed of growth, and the

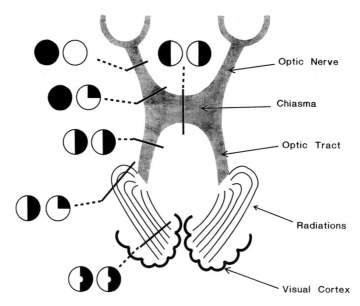

Fig. 6.22 *Visual field defects associated with lesions at various sites along the optic pathways.*

ability of the chiasma to distend can all have a significant effect upon the resultant field loss.

Tumours

The chiasma is one of the most vulnerable regions of the brain with respect to the development of tumours. While it is difficult to put exact figures on the percentage of brain tumours that arise from this region, several clinicians have estimated that it is around 25%.

There are three types of tumour commonly associated with chiasmal damage:

(a) An adenoma of the pituitary gland, which is by far the most common.
(b) A craniopharyngioma (tumour arising from the remnants of the craniopharygeal duct).
(c) A meningioma (tumour arising from the membranes covering the brain) (Greve and Raakman, 1977; Isayama, 1979).

It is also possible to get aneurysms of the neighbouring blood vessels that can exert pressure on the chiasma.

Pituitary tumours. The majority of pituitary adenomas are of the chromophobe (little affinity for dyes) type although other types, such as the eosinophilic (stain easily with eosin) and basophilic (stain readily with alkaline dyes), are occasionally found. In a study

of 66 pituitary adenomas, Isayama (1979) reported that 80% were chromophobe while the remaining 20% were eosinophilic.

As the chiasma lies approx. 10 mm above the roof of the pituitary fossa, it follows that a pituitary tumour must grow to a considerable size before it begins to compress the chiasma (see Figure 6.20). For this reason, patients with endocrine secreting tumours, such as the chromophilic adenomas, usually seek medical advice for the hormonal changes that occur before the tumour has reached a sufficient size to put any pressure on the chiasma and cause any visual field loss. Patients with non-secreting chromophobe adenomas often have visual field loss when they first seek medical advice (Spalton *et al.*, 1984).

The classic visual field defect associated with a pituitary tumour is a bitemporal hemianopia, starting with early loss in the upper temporal quadrant, gradually extending inferiorly to form a bitemporal hemianopia. If left unchecked, it continues round to involve the inferior nasal and finally the superior nasal fields (see Figure 6.23). The superior nasal field is the last to be affected due to the extreme lateral placement of these fibres within the chiasma. These field defects are often more apparent in the central isopters and are often relative rather than absolute (Isayama, 1979; Meinenberg *et al.*, 1985). The exact nature of the visual field loss is dependent upon the position of

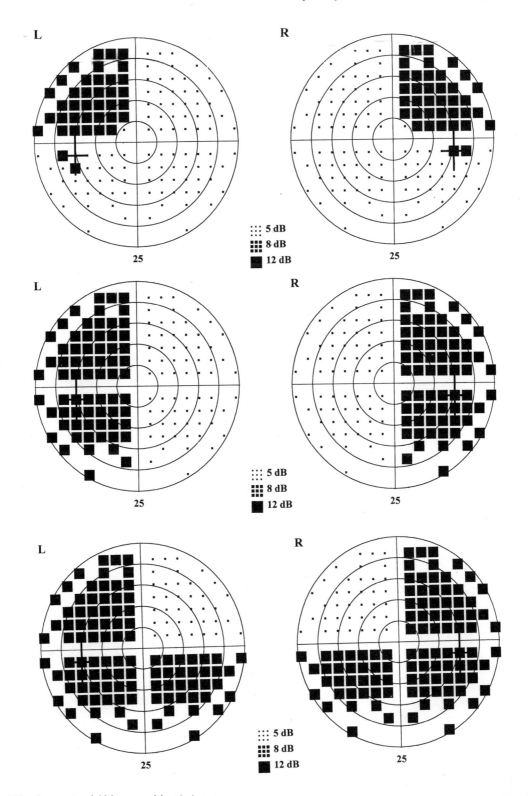

Fig. 6.23 *Progressive field loss caused by pituitary tumour.*

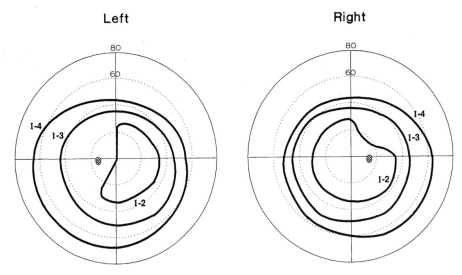

Fig. 6.24 *Bitemporal hemianopia affecting the central isopters.*

the tumour in relation to the chiasma. Normally, the tumour puts slightly more pressure on the anterior part of the chiasma and produces the sequence of field defects described above. If, however, the chiasma is prefixed, then the tumour will press more on the posterior part of the chiasma. The orthodox view is that pressure towards the posterior part of the chiasma produces bitemporal scotoma rather than bitemporal hemianopias. However, recent research is challenging this orthodox view.

A significant number of patients with pituitary tumours have atypical visual field defects such as unilateral central defects, unilaterally blind and bitemporal paracentral scotoma (Greve and Raakman, 1977; Isayama, 1979). Many of these are asymmetric and may only involve the central isopters (see Figure 6.24), although with time these may become more typical as the tumour enlarges. These atypical defects can easily lead to an incorrect diagnosis. Remember Murphy's law: if a field defect can be atypical it almost always is!

Another factor to consider with pituitary tumours is the direction in which the tumour is enlarging. If it puts more pressure towards one side of the chiasma then the resultant defects will show a large degree of right left asymmetry (see Figure 6.25).

With removal of the pituitary tumour there is a recovery of the visual field over a 1–2 month period, although this is rarely complete (Dannheim *et al.*,

1979). The extent of residual loss is dependent upon the degree of atrophy that has occurred.

Craniopharyngiomas and meningiomas. Craniopharyngiomas are tumours that arise from the remnants of the craniopharyngeal duct while meningiomas are tumours arising from the meninges. The types of defect associated with these tumours are very similar to those caused by pituitary tumours, although with meningiomas there is a larger number of asymmetric defects, including unilateral blindness, and bilateral and unilateral central defects (Greve and Raakman, 1977; Isayama, 1979).

THE OPTIC TRACTS

Anatomy

The two optic tracts leave the chiasma and proceed posteriorly and laterally to the lateral geniculate body (or nucleus) (see Figure 6.18). Before reaching the lateral geniculate, both tracts give off a branch – the brachium – which passes into the midbrain. This branch carries fibres relating to the control of eye movements and the pupil.

As the fibres pass towards the lateral geniculate those from corresponding regions of the right and left eyes become more and more closely associated.

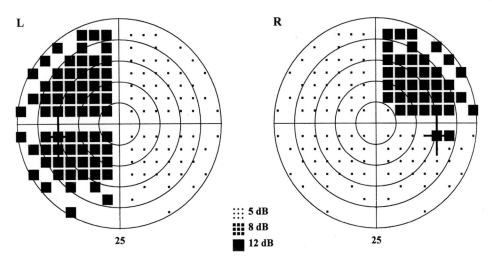

Fig. 6.25   *Asymmetric defect caused by pituitary tumour pressing on one side of the chiasma.*

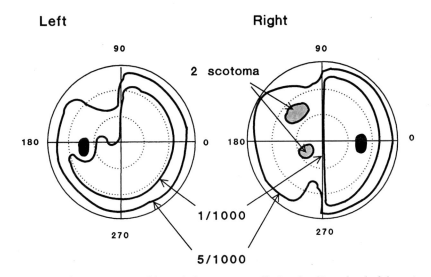

Fig. 6.26   *Left homonymous hemianopia caused by a pituitary tumour affecting the chiasmal end of the optic tract.*

Visual field defects associated with optic tract lesions

The position of the optic tracts, which are embedded in the cerebral hemispheres, makes the occurrence of an isolated tract lesion very rare. When other regions of the brain are involved the non-visual effects are invariably more obvious than the visual ones. Those isolated lesions that do occur are most often caused by pituitary tumours affecting the chiasmal end of the tracts. The ensuing defects will affect one hemifield, producing homonymous (a term which simply means

that it affects the same side) defects (see Figure 6.26). The defects also show large amounts of incongruity (different in each eye; see *Congruity*, pp. 65–66 for more comments on congruency).

THE LATERAL GENICULATE BODY
Anatomy

At the lateral geniculate body, the retinal ganglion cell fibres come to an end. Each ganglion cell axon

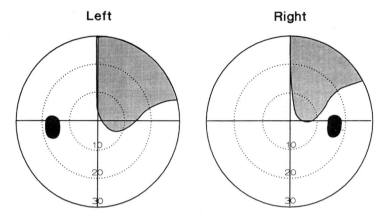

Fig. 6.27　*Right homonymous hemianopia caused by a lesion at the lateral geniculate body.*

synapses with a number of geniculate neurones, some of which project their axons to the visual cortex (geniculocortical cells), while others confine their connections to the lateral geniculate (interneurons).

The posterior aspect of the lateral geniculate, which contains fibres representing the central 15–20 degrees of the contralateral field, is composed of six layers. Each layer receives the ganglion cell fibres from only one eye: layers 1, 4 and 6 receive their input from the contralateral eye (other side) while layers 2, 3 and 5 receive their input from the ipsilateral eye (same side), i.e. the incoming fibres from the two eyes synapse on different geniculate layers.

In moving from the posterior to the anterior part of the lateral geniculate, layers 4 and 6 merge into a single layer, as do layers 3 and 5. The anterior aspect, which represents the peripheral field has four rather than six layers.

Each of the geniculate layers has a retinotopic map of the contralateral half of the visual field and each of these maps is in register with those from other layers. If you were to pass a recording electrode down through the different geniculate layers you would find, as you went from layer to layer, that the recorded responses all come from the same region of the visual field.

The exact reasons for the lateral geniculate being organized in this fashion is still the subject of a great deal of research. What is already known is that the cells within the dorsal four layers (3, 4, 5 and 6), which are called the parvocellular layers, are smaller than those in layers 1 and 2, the magnocellular layers, and that these two groups of cells have functional differences with

respect to the type of information they transmit. It appears, therefore, that the visual cells are divided at this level into different categories on the basis of the information they are carrying.

Visual field defects associated with lateral geniculate lesions

Damage to the lateral geniculate causes homonymous defects (affecting either the right or left field of both eyes, see Figure 6.27). However, the position of the lateral geniculate body makes it extremely rare for this structure to be involved in an isolated lesion. When neighbouring tissues are affected, the damage can often be so severe that it precludes any visual field examination.

OPTIC RADIATIONS
Anatomy

Axons from geniculate cells pass, in what is called the optic radiations, to the visual cortex. After leaving the lateral geniculate, the fibres ascend for a short distance before sweeping laterally and posteriorly towards the visual cortex. While the fibres from the medial aspect travel in an almost direct course to the visual cortex, those from the lateral aspect sweep anteriorly before looping round to then pass back to the visual cortex. This loop is known as Meyer's loop (see Figure 6.28). Its presence can have important implications with respect to localizing lesions, although again it must be stressed that there is a large amount of individual variability and the absence of a particular characteristic

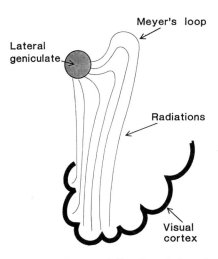

Fig. 6.28 *Course of the visual fibres from the lateral geniculate body to the visual cortex.*

cannot be used to exclude the possibility of the lesion being in a particular location.

Visual field defects associated with lesions to the optic radiations

Lesions to the optic radiations are normally vascular in origin and occur in patients who have generalized circulatory diseases such as arteriosclerosis. They normally have an abrupt appearance, which differentiates them from the slowly progressing defects associated with tumours.

Visual field defects that involve the optic radiations are normally confined to one hemisphere and produce visual field defects which are confined to one hemifield. Damage to the radiations on the right side of the brain cause visual field defects in the left field of both eyes and vice versa. The general rule, which applies to all lesions above the chiasma, is that the lesion lies on the opposite side to the visual field defects.

Lesions to the radiations also tend to be more congruous (alike in both eyes) than those of the optic tracts but less congruous than those from the visual cortex.

The nature of the visual field loss can be very helpful in localizing the site of a lesion.

Temporal lobe lesions
Temporal lobe lesions, which affect the radiations shortly after they have left the lateral geniculate, can produce what is known as a 'pie in the sky' field defect (see Figure 6.29). This is caused by the lesion selectively involving the fibres in Meyer's loop. Another characteristic of temporal lobe lesions is their tendency to split the macula. Lesions involving both the temporal and occipital lobes usually give rise to macular sparing (see *Macular sparing*, p. 66).

More posterior lesions
Lesions further back, towards the visual cortex, can often result in quadrantanopsias (loss of a quadrant). This is due to the continuing process of sorting and

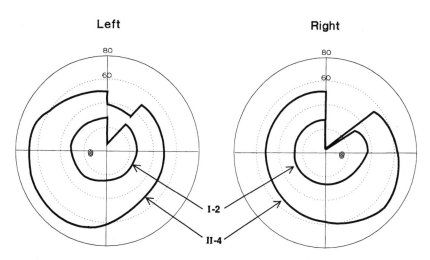

Fig. 6.29 *Field defect resulting from a lesion to the temporal lobe which damaged the optic radiations.*

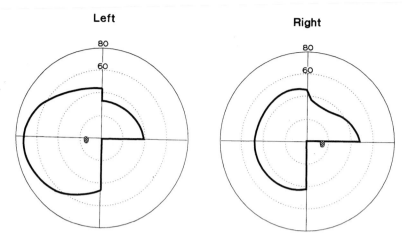

Fig. 6.30 *Quadrantanopsia caused by damage to the distal optic radiations.*

alignment that occurs along the visual pathways. Within the radiations there is a clear separation of the fibres emanating from the different regions of the visual field. Additionally, there is a separate blood supply to the dorsal and ventral fibres. The dorsal fibres are supplied by the middle cerebral artery which, if occluded, would produce an inferior quadrantanopsia (see Figure 6.30), while the lateral fibres are supplied by the posterior cerebral artery. As the posterior cerebral artery goes onto supply the visual cortex, occlusion of this vessel produces a complete homonymous hemianopia rather than a superior quadrantanopsia as would be predicted from a consideration of the radiations in isolation.

It should again be stressed that lesions to these regions of the brain often involve far more than the visual pathways and consequently there are numerous other localizing signs of the lesion.

THE VISUAL CORTEX
Anatomy
The cortex, a term which means rind or bark, is the outer 4–6 mm of the cerebrum, which itself is by far the largest part of the brain. The cortex is the 'grey matter' of the brain, a colour resulting from the very large number of nerve cells. The underlying white matter is composed of medullated nerve fibres on their way to and from different regions of the cortex (see Figure 6.31).

During embryonic development, the grey matter expands and forms numerous folds which give it the characteristic appearance with which we are all familiar (see Figure 6.31). The deeper folds are called fissures, while the shallower ones are called sulci. The cortex is divided into two hemispheres and into a number of different lobes. These divisions often follow the major fissures.

The visual cortex, that is the region of the cortex which receives the visual input from the eyes, lies in the occipital lobe, at the very back of the head. It has a particularly large fold in it known as the calcarine fissure.

The visual cortex is also known, after a numerical classification system devised by Brodmann, as area 17 and surrounding it are the parastriate region (Brodmann's area 18) and the peristriate region (Brodmann's area 19). There is no clear border between the parastriate and the peristriate regions and they are often grouped together and called the prestriate region.

Another common way of referring to the visual cortex is as the striate area. This name is derived from its appearance, the axons of the optic radiations forming a well-defined white line, known as the white line of Gennari.

If a recording electrode were systematically placed in different regions of the visual cortex then we would find that each region responded to stimuli presented over a small region of the visual field. There is a precise retinotopic map in each hemisphere of the opposite hemifield. The macular is projected over an area that is out of all proportion to its angular subtence. In fact, more than half of the striate cortex is devoted to the central 10 degrees of the visual field.

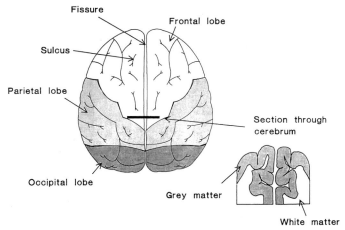

Fissure

Frontal lobe

Sulcus

Parietal lobe

Section through
cerebrum

Occipital lobe

Grey matter

White matter

Fig. 6.31 *Superior view of the cortex showing its major lobes.*

The visual cortex is composed of six different layers of nerve cells. The fibres from the lateral geniculate body, after passing through the radiations, predominantly terminate in layer 4. Those from the magnocellular layers of the lateral geniculate project mainly to the upper part of this layer while those from the parvocellular layers project mainly to the lower part of this layer. Other layers are associated with projections to other regions of the brain, such as the colliculus and the prestriate regions.

For a long time it was believed that the geniculate axons went solely to the striate cortex and from there connections were made to the prestriate regions. However, recent research has shown that there is a direct projection from the lateral geniculate to area 18. Area 18 thus receives two inputs from the lateral geniculate, one directly and the other via area 17.

Visual field defects associated with lesions to the visual cortex

There are three main causes of lesions to the visual cortex:

1. Vascular.
2. Tumours.
3. Trauma.

Vascular lesions

The majority of lesions affecting the visual cortex are vascular in origin, caused by arteriosclerosis of the posterior cerebral artery. The lesions are invariably confined to one hemisphere, producing homonymous defects which are perfectly congruent and often show macular sparing (see Figure 6.3). Patients will often report having had previous episodes of blurring or even blackouts, which are indicative of vascular insufficiency. The edges to the visual field defects are usually steep and there is little if any recovery.

Tumours

Another cause of lesions to the visual cortex is tumours. An obvious difference between this type of lesion and that produced by either trauma or vascular occlusions is its slow progression and gradual loss of visual field which progresses to a homonymous hemianopia. Neighbouring tissue is often affected giving rise to a large number of syndromes which together affect practically all the senses.

A tumour may interfere with the vascular supply, thereby mimicking a vascular lesion.

It has been reported that neoplasmic lesions tend to be less congruent than those caused by vascular lesions (Furuno, 1977).

Trauma

The diagnosis of trauma to the visual cortex is unambiguous. The resulting visual field defects are again homonymous, the extent being entirely dependent upon the amount and position of the damage. Traumatic lesions can affect both hemispheres, producing bilateral homonymous defects. Superior altitudinal defects are rare since damage to the corresponding region of the cortex invariably involves areas of the brain that are critical to survival. Loss of the field around the horizontal meridian is also rare, presumably because this region of the field is represented in the depths of the calcarine fissure, an area that is less likely to be involved in survivable trauma.

Some recovery of function is common during the healing process. This may be accompanied by the patient adopting extrafoveal fixation or even cyclorotation of the eyes in order to maximally benefit from any surviving field.

Macular sparing is far less common in trauma than in vascular lesions.

THE DIFFERENTIAL DIAGNOSIS OF VISUAL FIELD DEFECTS

Until now we have looked at the types of field defect that arise from lesions to a specific part of the primary visual pathways. While nobody would doubt that this is a very good way of dealing with this subject, it is not particularly helpful to the perimetrist who has just discovered a visual field defect and is wondering what could be causing it. This section is designed to help the perimetrist with this problem. It goes the other way, i.e. from the field defect to the likely pathology.

In the ideal world every pathology would have a unique type of visual field defect from which a diagnosis could confidently be made. Unfortunately this is not the case. While a given pathology may give rise to a certain type of defect this same defect could have arisen from a number of different pathologies. For example, toxic amblyopia produces a central/cecocentral defect. However, this same type of defect could have resulted from optic neuritis, toxic amblyopia, hereditary optic atrophy etc. In other words, a given type of defect does not necessarily have a good localizing value.

The three flow charts shown in Figures 6.32, 6.33 and 6.34 take you through a series of questions that eventually lead to a list of possible pathologies. The first question, 'Are there any ophthalmoscopic signs?' helps to simplify the diagrams. If every retinal condition which is likely to give rise to a visual field defect is included then, understandably, the flow charts become over-complex.

In using these flow charts care must be exercised not to exclude conditions that can occasionally mimic

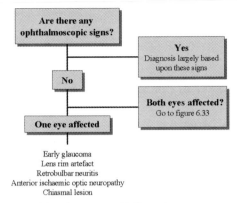

Fig. 6.32 *Flow diagram to aid diagnosis*

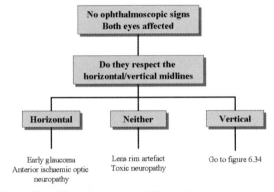

Fig. 6.33 *Flow diagram to aid diagnosis.*

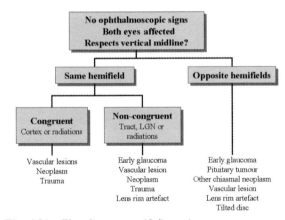

Fig. 6.34 *Flow diagram to aid diagnosis.*

other conditions. For example, glaucoma normally affects one eye before the other and retains some right–left asymmetry throughout its course, but there is a possibility that the two eyes will have similar-looking defects. Similarly, glaucoma normally produces defects that respect the horizontal midline. There is, however, always a chance that the defect will affect both the superior and inferior fields.

The list of pathologies given in each of the flow charts starts with the most common ones and proceeds to the less and less likely. This ranking should not, however, be taken too literally. Some practitioners may have more or less lens rim artefacts than others!

In providing these lists of pathologies I have also elected to generalize rather than be specific, e.g. 'neoplasm' appears instead of a long list of all the different types of tumour. This is justified on the grounds that it is not possible to differentiate between the different types of neoplasm on the basis of the visual field results.

REFERENCES

Aulhorn E. and Tanzil M. (1979) Comparison of visual field defects in glaucoma and in acute anterior ischemic optic neuropathy. *Doc Ophthalmol Proc Series*, **19**, 73–79.

Birchall C.H., Harris G.S., Drance S.M. and Begg I.S. (1976) Visual field changes in branch retinal vein occlusions. *Arch Ophthalmol*, **94**, 747–754.

Boughman J.A. and Fishman G.A. (1983) A genetic analysis of retinitis pigmentosa. *Br J Ophthalmol*, **67**, 449–454.

Brazitikos P.D., Safran A.B., Simona F. and Zulauf M. (1990) Threshold perimetry in tilted disc syndrome. *Arch Ophthalmol*, **108**, 1698–1700.

Brusini P., Dal Mas P., Della Mea G., Tosoni C. and Lucci B. (1987) Centro-caecal field examination in chronic alcoholism. *Doc Ophthalmol Proc Series*, **49**, 639–644.

Dannheim F., Luedecke D. and Kuehne D. (1979) Visual fields before and after transnasal removal of a pituitary tumor. *Doc Ophthalmol Proc Series*, **19**, 4351.

Dorrell D. (1978) The tilted disc. *Br J Ophthalmol*, **62**, 16–20.

Drasdo N. (1989) Receptive field densities of the ganglion cells of the human retina. *Vis Res*, **29**, 985–988.

Ehlers N. (1975) Quadrant sparing of the macula. *Acta Ophthalmol*, **53**, 393–402.

Friedmann A.H., Gartner S. and Modi S.S. (1979) Drusen of the optic disc – a retrospective study in cadaver eyes. *Br J Ophthalmol*, **59**, 413–421.

Furuno F. (1977) Some aetiological aspects of homonymous hemianoptic scotoma. *Doc Ophthalmol Proc Series*, **14**, 303–313.

Glaser J.S. (1978) *Neuro-ophthalmology*. Harper and Row, Hagerstown.

Graham M.V. and Wakefield G.J. (1973) Bitemporal visual field defects associated with anomalies of the optic discs. *Br J Ophthalmol*, **57**, 307–314.

Greve E.L. and Raakman M. (1977) On atypical chiasmal visual field defects. *Doc Ophthalmol Proc Series*, **14**, 315–325.

Gutteridge I.F. and Cockburn D.M. (1981) Optic nerve head drusen: a correlation of clinical signs. *Aust J Optom*, **64**, 252–255.

Harms H. (1977) Visual field defects in diseases of the fasciculus opticus. *Doc Ophthalmol Proc Series*, **14**, 289–297.

Hart W.M. and Burde R.M. (1983) Three-dimensional topography of the central visual field: sparing of foveal sensitivity in macular disease. *Ophthalmology*, **90**, 1028–1038.

Hayreh S.S. and Podhajsky P. (1979) Visual field defects in anterior ischemic optic neuropathy. *Doc Ophthalmol Proc Series*, **19**, 53–71.

Hill D.N. and Griffiths J.D. (1970) The prognosis in retinal vein thrombosis. *Trans Ophthalmol Soc UK*, **90**, 309–322.

Isayama Y. (1979) Visual field defects due to tumors of the stella region. *Doc Ophthalmol Proc Series*, **19**, 27–42.

Johnson M.W. and Vine A.K. (1987) Hydroxychloroquine therapy in massive total doses without retinal toxicity. *Am J Ophthalmol*, **104**, 139–144.

Keltner J.L., Johnson C.A., Spurr J.O. and Beck R.W. (1993) Baseline visual field profile of optic neuritis, the experience of the optic neuritis treatment trial. *Arch Ophthalmol*, **111**, 231–234.

Lavin P.J.M. and Ellenberger C. (1989) Traquair's monocular hemianopic junction scotoma, a sign of progressive optic neuropathy. In *Perimetry Update 1988/89* (ed. Heijl A.). Kugler & Ghendini, Amsterdam, pp. 91–95.

Lorentzen S.E. (1966) Drusen of the optic disc – clinical and genetic study. *Acta Ophthalmol Suppl*, **90**, 1–179.

Massof R.W., Dagnelie G., Benzschawel T., Palmer R.W. and Finkelstein D. (1990) First order dynamics of visual field loss in retinitis pigmentosa. *Clin Vis Sci*, **5**, 1–26.

Meienberg O., Mattle H., Jenni A. and Flammer J. (1985) Quantitative versus semiquantitative perimetry in neurological disorders. *Doc Ophthalmol Proc Series*, **42**, 233–237.

Roh S., Noecker R.J., Schuman J.S., Hedges T.R., Weiter J.J. and Mattox C. (1998) Effect of optic nerve head drusen on nerve fiber layer thickness. *Ophthalmology*, **105**, 878–885.

Rohrschneider K., Glück R., Fendrich T., Burk R.O.W., Kruse F.E. and Völcker H.E. (1997) Macular sparing in patients with hemianopsia. Re-evaluated using static and kinetic fundus perimetry. In *Perimetry Update 1996/1997* (ed. Wall M. and Heijl A.). Kugler & Ghendini, Amsterdam, pp. 377–385.

Sanchez-Dalmau B., Goni F.J., Guarro M., Roig C. and Duch-Bordas F. (1991) Bilateral homonymous visual field defects as initial manifestation of multiple sclerosis. *Br J Ophthalmol*, **75**, 185–187.

Sergott R.C. and Brown M.J. (1988) Current concepts of the pathogenesis of optic neuritis associated with multiple sclerosis. *Surv Ophthalmol*, **33**, 108–116.

Smith J.L. (1962) Homonymous hemianopia: A review of 100 cases. *Am J Ophthalmol*, **54**, 616–622.

Smith C.G. and Richardson W.F.G. (1966) The course and distribution of arteries supplying the visual (striate) cortex. *Am J Ophthalmol*, **61**, 1391–1396.

Spalton D.J., Hitchins R.A. and Hunter P.A. (1984) *Atlas of Clinical Ophthalmology*. Gower Medical, London.

Trobe J.D., Lorber M.L. and Schlezinger N.S. (1973) Isolated homonymous hemianopia. *Arch Ophthalmol*, **89**, 377–381.

von Szily (1922) Cited in Dorrell, 1978.

Young S.E., Walsh F.B. and Knox D.L. (1976) The tilted disc syndrome. *Am J Ophthalmol*, **82**, 16–23.

7 Glaucoma

INTRODUCTION

Of all the conditions that give rise to visual field loss, glaucoma must surely be the most important. Its high prevalence, existing in approximately 1.2% of the population over the age of 40 (Tuck and Crick, 1998), lack of symptoms and often tragic prognosis, give it a unique status for the perimetrist.

What exactly is glaucoma? There are many different definitions of glaucoma but, fortunately, they differ primarily on the basis of emphasis rather than content. A hopefully non-contentious definition is: 'An eye condition in which damage occurs to the nerve fibres at and around the optic nerve head. The damaged nerve fibres eventually die and atrophy which is accompanied by characteristic changes in the ophthalmoscopic appearance of the optic nerve head (e.g. increased cupping of the disc and notching of the neural retinal rim) and changes to the visual field. Glaucoma is often, but not always, associated with a raised intra-ocular pressure.'

Primary and secondary glaucoma

Glaucoma can occur as a result of a pre-existing ocular disease such as anterior uveitis. In this condition, the secretion of inflammatory cells can lead to a blockage of the normal aqueous drainage routes and a subsequent increase in the intra-ocular pressure. The pressure increase then damages the nerve fibres at the optic nerve head. This type of glaucoma is called secondary glaucoma because it occurs after a predisposing ocular condition (see Figure 7.1).

There are many conditions which give rise to secondary glaucoma, yet in total they only account for around 5% of all glaucoma (see Kanski and

McAllister, 1989 for more details on secondary glaucoma). Although secondary glaucoma is a very serious condition, visual field examination has little if any role to play in its diagnosis. Patients are normally already under the care of an ophthalmologist who is both treating the antecedent condition and aware of the likelihood of secondary glaucoma. In addition, secondary glaucoma invariably gives rise to a raised intra-ocular pressure and as such can be reliably detected with a tonometer. The role of visual field investigation is, therefore, largely confined to assessing the degree of damage to the posterior segment.

The other 95% of patients with glaucoma have primary glaucoma. This condition occurs without any antecedent ocular disease in an otherwise, apparently, healthy eye and are of prime concern to the perimetrist.

Primary glaucoma and the role of the perimetrist

There are three different types of primary glaucoma: open angle, closed angle and congenital (Figure 7.1). By far the most prevalent is primary open angle glaucoma, which accounts for approximately 66% of cases, while closed angle accounts for 33% and congenital 1%.

While these three conditions are all called primary glaucoma their aetiology is entirely different.

Congenital glaucoma is caused by a malformation of the aqueous drainage route from the eye thereby leading to a raised intra-ocular pressure.

Closed angle glaucoma is caused by the iris bulging forward and blocking the aqueous drainage route again leading to a raised intra-ocular pressure.

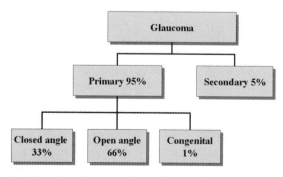

Fig. 7.1 *Classification and prevalence of glaucoma.*

The causes of open angle glaucoma are still not fully understood. In certain cases the intra-ocular pressure is raised and the mechanism of damage is similar to that of closed angle glaucoma. In other cases there is no evidence of there ever having been a raised intra-ocular pressure.

For the perimetrist there are important differences between these three types of primary glaucoma. Perimetry has, for obvious reasons, no practical role to play in the detection of congenital glaucoma and its role in closed angle glaucoma is largely restricted to assessing the degree of damage caused by the acute attacks. The severe symptoms and other ocular signs of closed angle glaucoma (blocked angle of anterior chamber, raised intra-ocular pressure, hazy cornea and fixed vertically oval pupil) makes it possible to diagnose this condition without recourse to a visual field examination.

Visual field examination does, however, feature prominently in both the diagnosis and management of primary open angle glaucoma.

Primary open angle glaucoma

In its early stages, primary open angle glaucoma is asymptomatic and its diagnosis is largely based upon the existence of three clinical signs: ophthalmoscopic changes at the optic nerve head, raised intra-ocular pressure and characteristic visual field loss. Unfortunately, in the early stages of open angle glaucoma, none of these three signs can be relied upon to detect all cases. Subtle changes at the optic nerve head are very difficult to recognize or to differentiate from the wide range of normal disc appearances (Gloster, 1978; Sommer *et al.*, 1979). Intra-ocular pressure measurements are often well within the normal range (Daubs and Crick, 1980) and field defects may not be detected until considerable damage has already occurred (Quigley *et al.*, 1982, 1989).

The monitoring of diagnosed cases of open angle glaucoma also presents a number of difficulties. While treatment is largely confined to reducing the intra-ocular pressure by either surgical or medical means there is no safe pressure below which further damage to the visual system will not occur.

Of all the three signs associated with open angle glaucoma, visual field loss has a unique attribute. Visual fields are a measure of visual function and visual field defects are a measure of functional loss.

While a measure of the intra-ocular pressure or an evaluation of the optic nerve head may lead the clinician to suspect functional loss they are not, in themselves, a measure of that functional loss. If one accepts that the objective of the eye caring professions is to retain as much functional vision as possible, then clearly visual field measures have a very important role to play in meeting that objective.

GLAUCOMATOUS FIELD DEFECTS

The following discussion of glaucomatous visual field defects begins with a description of their general characteristics, i.e. their location, size and evolution. It will then go on to discuss specific topics such as the relationship between focal and generalized loss and the degree of asymmetry between the right and left eyes. These are very important to the perimetrist as they often give key supportive evidence to a tentative diagnosis.

While the majority of what follows is based on results from patients with open angle glaucoma, field defects arising from acute attacks of closed angle glaucoma will be similar. The exception to this are the bizarre effects sometimes found with closed angle glaucoma such as loss of central vision (Reed and Drance, 1972).

Characteristics of glaucomatous visual field loss

The types of visual field loss associated with glaucoma are as follows:

1. paracentral,
2. arcuate,
3. nasal step,
4. overall depression,
5. baring of the blind spot,
6. enlargement of the blind spot.

Most of the defects occur within the central 30 degrees although the peripheral field is frequently involved (Stewart and Schields, 1991). For further discussion on the implications of confining visual field investigation to the central field, the reader is referred to Chapter 8.

Before getting involved in the details of these different types of visual field loss there is an important caveat that readers need to take on board.

While the field defects associated with glaucoma most often occur in certain regions of the field they are not confined to these regions. **Glaucomatous visual field defects can occur anywhere**.

The visual field defects falling in groups 1, 2 and 3 are collectively known as nerve fibre bundle defects and while the existence of one of these defects often indicates the presence of glaucoma they can arise from a number of other pathological conditions, such as anterior ischaemic optic neuropathy, optic nerve drusen, congenital pits and colobomas of the optic nerve head.

Paracentral defects

This type of defect, examples of which are shown in Figures 7.2 and 7.3, is frequently found in the early stages of glaucoma, approximately 70% of all early defects have a paracentral defect (Aulhorn and Harms, 1967). They occur more frequently in the superior rather than the inferior field, are more common in the arcuate areas (between 10 and 20 degrees of eccentricity) and are only rarely found at the macular or in the inferior temporal region (see Figure 7.4). These defects respect the nerve fibre distribution within the retina (see Chapter 6 on anatomy and pathologies of the visual pathways) in that they tend to follow the course of the nerve fibres and often show abrupt changes when they meet the horizontal midline. It is not unusual for there to be more than one paracentral defect although in the early stages they tend to be confined to either the superior or the inferior field (Hart and Becker, 1982; Mickelberg and Drance, 1984).

When plotted with kinetic techniques, these defects are often shown as having sharp edges and smooth contours. When plotted with static techniques the defects are found to have irregular borders and to demonstrate a good deal of variability from one session to another (see *Variability of field loss*, pp. 100–101). A large amount of variability should, therefore, make the perimetrist suspicious that a defect is present.

Arcuate defects

This type of defect represents a more advanced stage of glaucomatous visual field loss. It is often viewed as a coalition of a group of paracentral defects (see Figure 7.5). As the name implies, these defects lie in the

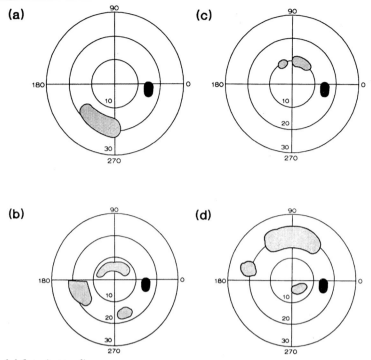

Fig. 7.2 *Paracentral defects, isopter diagrams.*

arcuate, or Bjerrum, regions above and/or below the macular often extending from the horizontal midline to the disc. These defects, like the paracentral defects, are more often found in the superior rather than the inferior field. They respect the horizontal midline and again, when kinetically plotted, are often represented as smooth-edged defects. Static instruments show a more irregular pattern and significant amounts of variability from one session to another (see Figure 7.3).

Nasal step

Nasal step is a characteristic defect associated with a difference in the sensitivity above and below the horizontal midline in the nasal field. This sensitivity difference, when investigated with a kinetic strategy, gives rise to a 'step' in the isopter (see Figure 7.6). The sensitivity loss associated with this type of defect is more frequent in the superior field (Hart and Becker, 1982).

It is important to realize that small steps are not uncommon in normal patients. It is only when these steps exceed a certain value that they are considered significant. The critical value, differentiating normal from suspicious, has not been clearly defined, although it varies with eccentricity being greater in the periphery than in the central field (Drance *et al.*, 1979). Most published examples cite steps of around 5–10 degrees as significant.

The existence of a nasal step is a particularly valuable sign for several reasons. It occurs in a large percentage of patients with glaucomatous loss (up to 40%, Caprioli and Spaeth, 1985) and it is highly specific to glaucoma. (There are other conditions that affect the optic nerve head that may also give rise to nasal steps.) In addition to this, its known location means that the perimetrist only needs a few moments to establish its presence.

While nasal step occurs in a large percentage of cases with early field loss, it is rarely seen in isolation. The exact percentage of patients who have an isolated nasal step varies from one report to another. Aulhorn and Harms (1967) report that it occurs in only 0.7% of patients; Armaly (1971) reports that it occurs in 1.9%, LeBlanc and Becker (1971) in 11%, Drance *et al.* (1979) in 20% and LeBlanc *et al.* (1985) in 0%. These differences most likely result from the use of

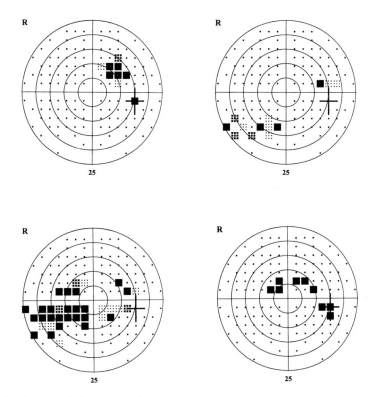

Fig. 7.3 *Paracentral and arcuate defects, grey scale.*

different techniques of investigation, and different definitions of clinically significant nasal step.

The static correlate of nasal step would be a difference in the sensitivity above and below the horizontal midline. Jenni *et al.* (1989) specifically looked for this in a group of normal and glaucomatous patients. They used a full threshold strategy to compare the sensitivity of four pairs of test points located above and below the horizontal midline in the central nasal field. While their results demonstrated that the suspect group had a greater variance of results, the overall variability in individual sensitivity measures reduced the value of this type of analysis to a level where it gave little, if any, additional information beyond that obtained with the index of corrected loss variance (see Chapter 9 for a definition of corrected loss variance). A more significant result might have been found if the researchers had looked in the peripheral field where the incidence of nasal step and the extent of the sensitivity difference is more pronounced (LeBlanc *et al.*, 1985).

Overall depression

Overall depression, as the name implies, is a gradual sinking of the island of vision resulting in reduced sensitivity measures and a contraction of isopters. This type of defect is very different to the focal lesions described above, which result from damage to specific nerve fibre bundles at the optic nerve head. Overall depression is believed to be the result of a diffuse loss of nerve fibres throughout the optic nerve. Its existence has been noted to occur in up to 38% of patients with glaucomatous loss (Aulhorn and Harms, 1967; Armaly, 1971; Hart and Becker, 1982). It is, however, not specific to glaucoma. Changes to the crystalline lens (cataracts) cause a similar overall depression, as do the normally occurring age changes in the retina. Hart and Becker (1982) noted that while this defect can often be detected in retrospective studies, its existence contributes little to diagnosis.

Depression of the nasal field with contraction of just the nasal isopters, analogous to a listing of the island of vision (see Figure 7.7), is more specific to glaucoma and has also been noted to occur in a high proportion of cases (Rassi and Schields, 1982; Caprioli and Spaeth, 1985).

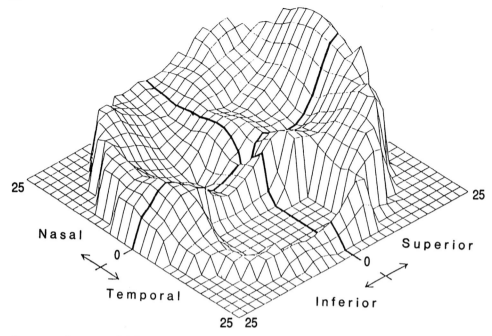

Fig. 7.4 *Frequency of paracentral defects in primary glaucoma.*

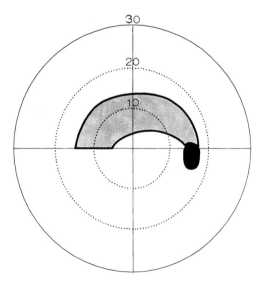

Fig. 7.5 *Superior arcuate defect, result from kinetic examination.*

Baring of the blind spot

This type of field defect is often associated with glaucoma, although its importance in both differential diagnosis and detection of glaucoma has been questioned. It results from a sensitivity difference above and below the disc, the area below the disc invariably being a little more sensitive than that above the disc. When the field is plotted kinetically with a stimulus whose intensity is set to be just above that of the retinal threshold below the disc, then it is not unusual to plot an isopter that curves around the disc (see Figure 7.8). This type of defect is called baring of the blind spot because the isopter no longer includes the disc. While this type of defect is found in glaucoma patients, often as part of an arcuate defect, it is no longer considered to be specific to glaucoma. It is possible, provided the correct stimulus is chosen, to bare the blind spot in normal patients. It should also be remembered that the sensitivity of the eye decreases with age and an isopter that formerly included the disc might, on subsequent examination, bare the disc purely as a result of normal age changes.

Enlargement of the blind spot

There are many different pathologies which can give rise to an enlarged blind spot. When enlargement is due to glaucoma it is usually in the form of an elongation along the course of the nerve fibres (Reed and

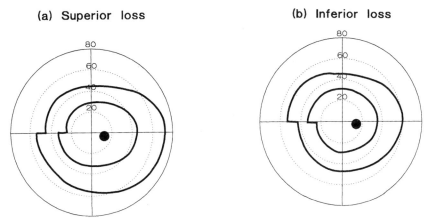

Fig. 7.6 *Nasal steps due to superior (a) and inferior (b) sensitivity loss.*

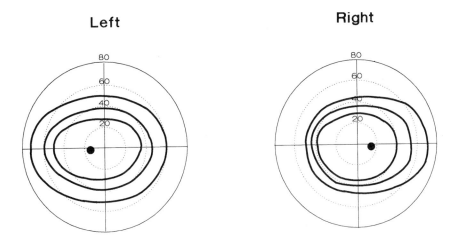

Fig. 7.7 *Depression of right nasal field with resulting contraction of nasal isopters.*

Drance, 1978). While this type of defect has been report in a relatively high proportion of glaucoma cases (Hart and Becker, 1982, reported it to exist in 55% of early cases), it is no longer believed to have much value in the early diagnosis of the disease. It is only rarely found in isolation and is difficult to differentiate from the normal disc, which shows a wide range of different sizes and shapes.

Classification with artificial neural network

The classification of glaucomatous visual field defects given in the previous sections is subjective, i.e. it is based on reviews of clinical data. Subjective classifications have a number of shortcomings:

1. The individual classes often lack precise definitions, e.g. when does a paracentral defect become and arcuate defect.
2. Small number of classes. This shortcoming is particularly relevant to the problems associated with the monitoring of glaucomatous loss when ideally progression could be defined on the basis of when the defect progresses from one class to the next.
3. The classification is based upon preconceived notions concerning the nature of glaucomatous loss that may not be correct.

In an attempt to overcome these problems Henson, Spenceley *et al.* (1996) utilized an artificial neural

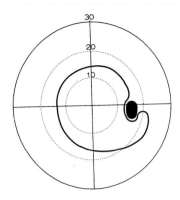

Fig. 7.8 *Baring of the blind spot.*

network known as a Kohonen self-organizing feature map to classify glaucomatous visual field defects. The network creates its classes from looking at a large number of glaucomatous visual field defects. It is looking for common spatial patterns of loss. Henson, Spenceley *et al.*, (1996) classified the superior and inferior hemifield separately and gave 25 patterns of loss for each hemifield (see Figure 7.9). The 25 classes were arranged in a two-dimensional map in which similar classes were adjacent to each other while the extreme classes (normal and blind) are at opposite ends of the map. This type of arrangement has potential for monitoring progressive loss (see Henson *et al.*, 1997).

Evolution of glaucomatous field defects

Even when treated, patients with glaucoma can continue to lose their visual field (Hart and Becker, 1982; Mickelberg and Drance, 1984; Katz, Gilbert *et al.* 1996). While the classic view is that those patients with more advanced field loss show an accelerated rate of progression (Wilson *et al.*, 1982; Mickelberg *et al.*, 1986), some recent work has concluded that rate is independent of the extent of loss (Katz, Gilbert *et al.*, 1996). Clearly, there are many issues that could explain these different findings, an important one being the nature of the treatment. Recent developments in glaucoma therapy mean that IOPs can often be maintained at lower values than was hitherto possible.

Progressive loss of the visual field can take place in a number of different ways:

(a) linear, increasing at a constant rate;

(b) curvilinear, increasing at a rate which itself increases with scotoma mass;

(c) episodic, there being periods of rapid progression and periods of relative stability (Mickelberg *et al.*, 1986).

When it comes to predicting the long-term extent of damage, which is important when assessing likely outcomes, McNaught *et al.*, (1995) have demonstrated that linear models are the most precise.

It has been suggested that the earliest sign of glaucomatous loss is an increased scatter of responses in an area that subsequently develops a defect. Another early sign is a slight asymmetry between the two eyes. This may manifest itself as a difference in the positions of the isopters or as a difference in the mean sensitivities. These changes, which may in themselves be intermittent, eventually lead to more specific defects such as a nasal step or a paracentral scotoma. These defects then enlarge and deepen but are often confined to either the superior or inferior field. In some patients the entire superior field may have been destroyed before the second hemifield becomes involved.

Focal loss and generalized loss

The defects associated with open angle glaucoma can be classified as either focal, in which the damage occurs to a specific bundle of nerve fibres, or generalized, in which it occurs to the whole optic nerve. Focal defects (paracentral and arcuate scotomas) are relatively deep and correspond to the nerve fibre distribution within the optic nerve head. Generalized loss is a small but significant loss in sensitivity across the whole visual field characterized by isopter contraction and a reduced mean sensitivity. This classification of defects into two categories has led some researchers to propose that there are two separate mechanisms associated with glaucomatous loss (Flammer *et al.*, 1985). One gives rise to focal loss while the other gives rise to generalized loss.

While some early results from full threshold perimetry brought into question the existence of diffuse loss (Heijl 1989; Åsman and Heijl, 1994), later work (Henson *et al.*, 1999) has demonstrated that it is a common accompanying feature of early glaucoma. It is, however, relatively rare for diffuse loss to exist without some localized loss (Drance *et al.*, 1987; Chauhan *et al.*, 1997).

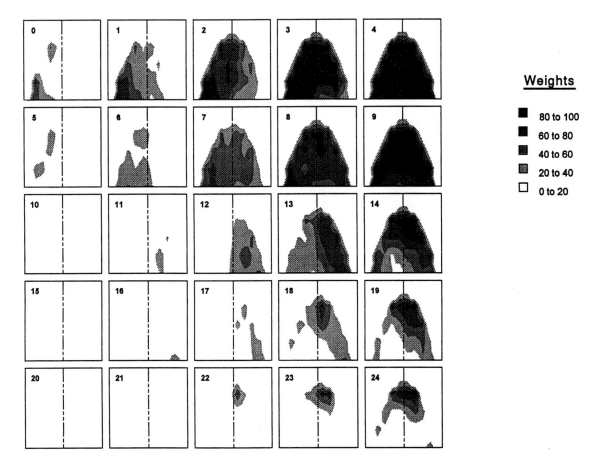

Weights

- ■ 80 to 100
- ■ 60 to 80
- ▨ 40 to 60
- ▥ 20 to 40
- □ 0 to 20

Fig. 7.9 *Classification of glaucomatous visual field defect found in the superior hemifield with an Artificial Neural Network. The network has organized the classes in a square matrix with the most advanced class in the top right hand corner and normal eyes in the bottom left.*

Asymmetry of field defects

While glaucoma is invariably a bilateral condition (involving both the right and left eyes), its progression is often asymmetric, occurring in one eye before the other and, when both eyes are involved, being more advanced in one eye compared to the other (see Figure 7.10). These asymmetries are not confined to visual field measures but also occur in measures of the intra-ocular pressure and the ophthalmoscopic appearance of the optic nerve head. The recognition of this asymmetry, which has been reported to occur in over 90% of glaucomatous cases (Henson *et al.*, 1986; Sponsel *et al.*, 1987) has led researchers to query whether such asymmetry could be useful in the early diagnosis of glaucoma (Lichter and Standardi, 1979).

An analysis of the results from full threshold techniques has shown that in normal patients asymmetries between the two eyes rarely exceed the differences found on repeat testing of the same eye (Feuer and Anderson, 1989). Feuer and Anderson suggest that mean differences (see Chapter 9 on quantification for details of how this is derived) of 2 dB on a single measure should be viewed with suspicion. Care should be exercised to ensure that alternative explanations, such as early changes in the crystalline lens, do not account for the measured differences. In summary, asymmetries in mean sensitivity should be viewed as a helpful corroborative sign, while in isolation they should make the clinician suspicious enough to warrant further investigation.

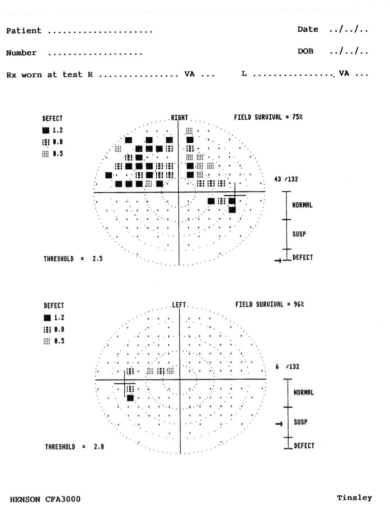

Fig. 7.10 *Glaucomatous visual field defect showing a large amount of asymmetry between the right and left eyes.*

In addition to the asymmetries between the two eyes, there is frequently an asymmetry between the superior and inferior hemifields (Hart and Becker, 1982; Mickelberg and Drance, 1984; Duggan *et al.*, 1985). This type of asymmetry forms the basis of the glaucoma hemifield test (Åsman and Heijl, 1992) of the Humphrey Visual Field Analyzer. This test has been shown to be an extremely reliable method for the detection of visual field loss (Katz, Quigley *et al.*, 1996). (For more details on the glaucoma hemifield test see Chapter 9 on quantification).

Variability of field loss
Patients with glaucoma demonstrate an increase in the

variability of their responses. This increase is related to sensitivity (see Chapter 2, section 7.1); the lower the sensitivity the greater the variability. In patients with localized loss variability will be high at and around the visual field defect while being relatively low at test locations where the sensitivity is normal.

Figure 7.11 gives the results from a Humphrey 24–2 full-threshold test on a patient with a large superior glaucomatous visual field defect. The Humphrey instrument repeats threshold estimates at certain locations and prints the repeat values, in brackets, underneath the first estimate. What can be seen in this figure is that in areas of normal sensitivity, below the fixation point, repeat estimates give similar values to the first estimate. However, in areas where there is a relative defect, below the blind spot and the extreme nasal field, just below the horizontal midline, repeat measures give very different threshold estimates. Below the blind spot the threshold reduces from 10 to <0 dB while in the inferior nasal field it decreases from 12 to 4 dB.

Detecting glaucomatous loss

Increased variability has been recognized for some time as being one of the earliest signs of glaucomatous damage. In a recent study by Heijl, in which he looked at the time it takes for a patient to convert from being normal to glaucomatous, normal being defined as three consecutive normal visual field results while glaucomatous was defined as three consecutive abnormal visual field results (normality being based upon the glaucoma hemifield test, see Chapter 9, p. 125), Heijl found that, on average, it takes 3.5 years to convert, i.e. for 3.5 years the patient is giving threshold results that keep changing between normal and abnormal. For more details on techniques for detecting glaucomatous loss see Chapter 9.

Monitoring loss

The increased variability seen at locations with reduced sensitivity creates an even bigger problem when it comes to deciding whether or not a visual field defect has progressed. The edges of defects and areas of localized loss, where change is most likely to occur, are exactly those locations that show the greatest variability. There is a danger that a sudden apparent change in the visual field will result in an unnecessary therapeutic change.

Theories

The causes of this increased variability are at present unknown, although various suggestions have been made:

1. due to a reduction in the density of ganglion cells (Wall *et al.*, 1997);
2. due to an increased susceptibility to fatigue (Donovan *et al.*, 1978);
3. due to poor fixation control (Henson, Evans *et al.*, 1996).

Currently, the most attractive theory is that relating it

to the density of ganglion cells. This theory can explain the increased variability seen in the peripheral field of normal patients, the increased variability seen in pathologies other than glaucoma (Henson *et al.* 2000) and the decreased variability seen with increased stimulus size (Wall *et al.*, 1997).

Solution

What is the solution to the increased variability seen in glaucoma? At present the only solution is to repeat the measurement. Repeat measures will help to differentiate between random variations in the visual field and true change. In a condition where the rate of change is often slow it has been suggested that at least six measures of the visual field are necessary before significant change can be differentiated from random noise. The cost implications of this to a glaucoma service are considerable and there is a great deal of activity currently taking place to try to develop better techniques for monitoring glaucoma which are subject to less variability.

DIFFERENCES BETWEEN NORMAL-TENSION AND HIGH-TENSION GLAUCOMA

Primary open angle glaucoma can be classified, on the basis of intra-ocular pressure measures, into:

(a) normal-tension glaucoma;
(b) high-tension glaucoma.

While a generally accepted definition of normal-tension glaucoma is 'a progressive visual field loss of a glaucomatous nature in conjunction with normal intra-ocular pressure', there is no general agreement on the cut-off value between high and normal-tension glaucoma.

Normal-tension glaucoma accounts for up to 30% of all open angle glaucoma and produces a particularly awkward problem for the ophthalmologist whose standard form of treatment is to reduce the intra-ocular pressure. If the pressure is not high is there any value in reducing it? The data of Crichton *et al.*, (1989) and the results from the collaborative normal-tension glaucoma study (Collaborative Normal-Tension Glaucoma Study Group, 1998) indicate that at least a percentage of these patients will benefit from pressure-reducing therapy.

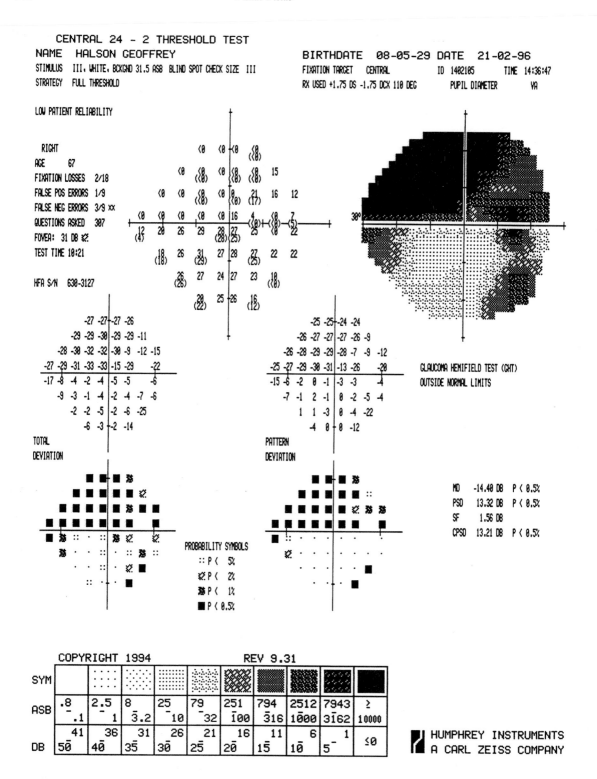

Fig. 7.11 *Humphrey visual field chart showing a glaucomatous eye with a superior arcuate defect. Note from the sensitivity values (top left map) that repeat measures (in brackets), in areas of relative loss, are subject to a large amount of variability.*

An interesting question concerning both high- and normal-tension glaucoma that has been asked by several independent groups of researchers, is whether there are any differences in the type of field loss in these two types of glaucoma?

Early studies, which were largely based upon manual perimetry, often gave equivocal results. Some researchers reported that low-tension glaucoma defects were closer to the fixation point and had steeper gradients (Levene, 1980; Hitchins and Anderton, 1983; Caprioli and Spaeth, 1984) while others reported that there were no differences, (Motolko *et al.*, 1982; Greve and Geijssen, 1983; Phelps *et al.*, 1983; King *et al.*, 1986).

In 1987 Drance conducted an investigation among patients in whom only one hemifield was affected with focal loss (Drance *et al.*, 1987). They wished to establish whether or not there were any differences in the sensitivities of the spared hemisphere between patients with high-tension and low-tension glaucoma. They found that there was twice as much sensitivity loss in the patients with high-tension glaucoma, a finding which supports the hypothesis that there is more diffuse loss in patients with high-tension glaucoma.

In a paper by Chauhan *et al.*, (1989), in which low-tension and high-tension glaucoma patients were carefully matched for the extent of damage, as expressed by the index mean deviation, patients with high-tension glaucoma were found to have significantly less normal test locations than those with low-tension glaucoma. This result again supports the hypothesis that there is more diffuse damage to the visual field in high-tension glaucoma. It must be emphasized, however, that these differences can only be found when the results from many patients are averaged; there will be many instances when low-tension patients are found to have diffuse damage and high-tension patients are found to have focal damage.

CONCLUSION

There is no doubt that visual field measures have a very important role to play in the detection and management of glaucoma. At the detection stage visual field strategies can be designed which are both highly sensitive and specific to glaucomatous loss, while at the management stage different strategies can be used to estimate the degree of functional loss

and whether any treatment has been successful. Remember the *raison d'être* of treatment is the preservation of visual function.

REFERENCES

Armaly M.F. (1971) Visual field defects in early open angle glaucoma. *Trans Am Ophthalmol Soc*, **69**, 147–162.

Åsman P. and Heijl A. (1992) Glaucoma hemifield test. Automated visual field evaluation. *Arch Ophthalmol*, **110**, 812–819.

Åsman P. and Heijl A. (1994) Diffuse visual field loss and glaucoma. *Acta Ophthalmol*, **72**, 303–308.

Aulhorn E. and Harms H. (1967) Early visual field defects in glaucoma. In *Glaucoma Symposium: Tutzing Castle.* Karger, Basle, pp. 151–186.

Armaly M.F. (1977) Selective perimetry for glaucomatous defects in ocular hypertension. *Arch Ophthalmol*, **87**, 518–524.

Caprioli J. and Spaeth G.L. (1984) Comparison of visual field defects in the low-tension glaucomas with those in high-tension glaucoma. *Am J Ophthalmol*, **97**, 730–737.

Caprioli J. and Spaeth G.L. (1985) Static threshold estimation of the peripheral nasal field in glaucoma. *Arch Ophthalmol*, **103**, 1150–1154.

Chauhan B.C., Drance S.M., Douglas G.R. and Johnson C.A. (1989) Visual field in normal-tension and high-tension glaucoma. *Am J Ophthalmol*, **108**, 636–642.

Chauhan B.C., LeBlanc R.P., Shaw A.M. *et al.*, (1997) Repeatable diffuse visual field loss in open-angle glaucoma. *Ophthalmology*, **104**, 532–538.

Collaborative Normal-Tension Glaucoma Study Group (1998) Comparison of glaucomatous progression between untreated patients with normal-tension glaucoma and patients with therapeutically reduced intra-ocular pressure. *Am J Ophthalmol*, **126**, 487–497.

Crichton A., Drance S.M., Douglas G.R. and Schultzer M. (1989) Unequal intra-ocular pressure and its relation to asymmetric visual field defects in low tension glaucoma. In *Perimetry Update 1988/89* (ed. Heijl A.). Kugler & Ghedini, Amsterdam, pp. 269–272.

Daubs J. and Crick R.P. (1980) Epidemiological analysis of King's College Hospital glaucoma data. *Res Clin Forums*, **2**, 41–59.

Donovan H.C., Weale R.A. and Wheeler C. (1978) The perimeter as a monitor of glaucomatous damage. *Br J Ophthalmol*, **62**, 705–708.

Drance S.M. (1969) The early field defects in glaucoma. *Invest Ophthalmol*, **8**, 84–91.

Drance S.M. (1972) The glaucomatous field. *Invest Ophthalmol*, **11**, 85–97.

Drance S.M., Douglas G.R., Airaksinen P.J., Schultzer M. and Hitchins R.A. (1987) Diffuse visual field loss in chronic open-angle low-tension glaucoma. *Am J Ophthalmol*, **104**, 577–580.

Drance S.M., Fairclough M., Thomas B., Douglas G.R. and Susanna R. (1979) The early visual field defect in glaucoma and the significance of nasal steps. *Doc Ophthalmol Proc Series*, **19**, 119–126.

Duggan C., Sommer A., Auer C. and Burkhard K (1985) Automated differential threshold perimetry for detecting glaucomatous visual field loss. *Am J Ophthalmol*, **100**, 420–423.

Feuer W.J. and Anderson D.R. (1989) Static threshold asymmetry in early glaucomatous visual field loss. *Ophthalmology*, **96**, 1285–1297.

Flammer J., Drance S.M. and Fankhauser F. (1984) Differential light threshold in automated static perimetry. *Arch Ophthalmol*, **102**, 876–879.

Flammer J., Drance S.M. and Zulaf M. (1984) Differential light threshold short and long-term fluctuations in patients with glaucoma, normal controls and patients with suspected glaucoma. *Arch Ophthalmol*, **102**, 704–706.

Flammer J., Drance S.M., Augustine L. and Funkhouser A. (1985) Quantification of glaucomatous visual field defects with automated perimetry. *Invest Ophthalmol Vis Sci*, **26**, 176–181.

Gloster J. (1978) Quantitative relationship between cupping of the optic disc and visual field loss in chronic simple glaucoma. *Br J Ophthalmol*, **65**, 665–669.

Greve E.L. and Geijssen H.C. (1983) Comparison of glaucomatous visual field defects in patients with high and low intra-ocular pressure. *Doc Ophthalmol Proc Series*, **35**, 101–105.

Hart W.M. and Becker B. (1982) The onset and evolution of glaucomatous visual field defects. *Ophthalmology*, **89**, 268–279.

Heijl A. (1989) Lack of diffuse loss in differential light sensitivity in early glaucoma. *Acta Ophthalmol*, **67**, 353–360.

Heijl A. and Drance S.M. (1983) Changes in differential threshold in patients with glaucoma during prolonged perimetry. *Br J Ophthalmol*, **67**, 512–516.

Henson D.B. and Bryson H. (1991) Is the variability in glaucomatous field loss due to poor fixation control? In *Perimetry Update 1990/91* (eds Mills P. and Heijl A.). Kugler, Amsterdam, pp. 217–220.

Henson D.B. and Hobley A.J. (1986) Frequency distribution of early glaucomatous visual field defects. *Am J Optom Physiol Optics*, **63**, 455–461.

Henson D.B., Artes P.H. and Chauhan B.C. (1999) Diffuse loss of sensitivity in early glaucoma. *Invest Ophthalmol Vis Sci*, **40**, 3147–3151.

Henson D.B., Evans J., Chauhan B.C. and Lane C. (1996) Influence of fixation accuracy on threshold variability in patients with open angle glaucoma. *Invest Ophthalmol Vis Sci*, **37**, 444–450.

Henson D., Hobley A., Chauhan B., Sponsel W. and Dallas N. (1986) Importance of visual field score asymmetry in the detection of glaucoma. *Am J Optom Physiol Optics*, **63**, 714–723.

Henson D.B., Spenceley S.E. and Bull D.R. (1996) Spatial classification of glaucomatous visual field loss. *Br J Ophthalmol*, **80**, 526–531.

Henson D.B., Spenceley S.E. and Bull D.R. (1997) Artificial neural network analysis of noisy visual field data in glaucoma. *Art Intelligence Med*, **10**, 99–113.

Henson D.B., Chaudry S., Artes P.H., Faragher E. B. and Ansons A. (2000) Response variability in the visual field: Comparison of optic neuritis, glaucoma, ocular hypertension and normal eyes. *Invert Ophthalmol Vis Sci*, **41**, 417–421.

Hitchins R.A. and Anderton S.A. (1983) A comparative study of visual field defects seen in patients with low-tension glaucoma and chronic simple glaucoma. *Br J Ophthalmol*, **67**, 818–821.

Jenni A., Hirsbrunner H.P. and Fankhauser F. (1989) The nasal step in the normal and glaucomatous visual field. In *Perimetry Update 1988/89* (ed. Heijl A.). Kugler and Ghedini, Amsterdam, pp. 305–311.

Katz J., Gilbert D., Quigley H.A. and Sommer A. (1996) Estimating progression of visual field loss in glaucoma. *Ophthalmology*, **104**, 1017–1025.

Katz J., Quigley H.A. and Sommer A. (1996) Detection of incident field loss using the glaucoma hemifield test. *Ophthalmology*, **103**, 657–663.

Kanski J.J. and McAllister J.A. (1989) *Glaucoma. A Colour Manual of Diagnosis and Treatment*. Butterworths, Sevenoaks.

King D., Drance S.M., Douglas G., Schultzer M. and Weijsman K. (1986) Comparison of visual field defects in normal-tension glaucoma and high-tension glaucoma. *Am J Ophthalmol*, **101**, 204–207.

Langerhorst C.T., Van Den Berg T.J.T.P. and Greve E. (1989) Fluctuation and general health in automated perimetry in glaucoma. In *Perimetry Update 1988/89* (ed. Heijl A.). Kugler and Ghedini, Amsterdam, pp.159–164.

LeBlanc R.P. and Becker B. (1971) Peripheral nasal field defects. *Am J Ophthalmol*, **72**, 415–419.

LeBlanc R.P., Lee A. and Baxter M. (1985) Peripheral nasal field defects. *Doc Ophthalmol Proc Series*, **42**, 377–381.

Levene R.Z. (1980) Low-tension glaucoma. A critical review and new material. *Surv Ophthalmol*, **24**, 621–664.

Lichter P.R. and Standardi C.L. (1979) Early glaucomatous visual field defects and their significance to clinical ophthalmology. *Doc Ophthalmol Proc Series*, **19**, 111–119.

McNaught A.I., Crabb D.P., Fitzke F.W. and Hitchins R.A. (1995) Modelling series of visual fields to detect progression in normal tension glaucoma. *Graef's Arch Clin Exp Ophthalmol*, **233**, 750–755.

Mickelberg F.S. and Drance S.M. (1984) The mode of progression of visual field defects in glaucoma. *Am J Ophthalmol*, **98**, 443–445.

Mickelberg F.S., Schultzer M., Drance S.M. and Lau W. (1986) The rate of progression of scotomas in glaucoma. *Am J Ophthalmol*, **101**, 1–6.

Motolko M., Drance S.M. and Douglas G.R. (1982) Comparison of defects in low-tension glaucoma and chronic open angle glaucoma. *Arch Ophthalmol*, **100**, 1074–1077.

Phelps C.D., Hayreh S.S. and Montague P.R. (1983) Visual field in low-tension glaucoma, primary open angle glaucoma, and anterior ischemic optic neuropathy. *Doc Ophthalmol Proc Series*, **35**, 113–124.

Quigley H.A., Addicks E.M. and Green W.R. (1982) Optic nerve damage in human glaucoma: III. Quantitative correlation of nerve fibre loss and visual field defect in glaucoma, ischemic neuropathy, and toxic neuropathy. *Arch Ophthalmol*, **100**, 135–146.

Quigley H.A., Dunkelberger G.R. and Green W.R. (1989) Retinal ganglion cell atrophy correlated with automated perimetry in human eyes with glaucoma. *Am J Ophthalmol*, **107**, 453–464.

Rassi M.O. and Schields M.B. (1982) Crowding of the peripheral nasal isopters in glaucoma. *Am J Ophthalmol*, **94**, 4–10.

Reed H. and Drance S.M. (1972) *The Essentials of Perimetry. Static and Kinetic*. Oxford University Press, Oxford.

Sommer A., Pollack I. and Maumenee A.E. (1979) Optic disc parameters and onset of glaucomatous field loss. I Methods and progressive change in disc morphology. *Arch Ophthalmol*, **97**, 1444–1448.

Sponsel W.E., Hobley A., Henson D.B., Chauhan B.C. and Dallas N.L. (1987) Quantitative supra-threshold static perimetry; the value of field score and asymmetry in the detection of chronic open angle glaucoma. *Doc Ophthalmol Proc Series*, **49**, 217–229.

Stewart W.C. and Shields M.B. (1991) The peripheral visual field in glaucoma: re-evaluation in the age of automated perimetry. *Surv Ophthalmol*, **36**, 59–69.

Tuck M.W. and Crick R.P. (1998) The age distribution of primary open angle glaucoma. *Ophthalmic Epidemiol*, **5**, 173–183.

Vingrys A.J. and Verbaken J.H. (1990) Perimetric fluctuation in diseased eyes. ARVO, abstract no. 1296.

Wall M., Kutzo K.E. and Chauhan B.C. (1997) Variability in patients with glaucomatous visual field damage is reduced using size V stimuli. *Invest Ophthalmol Vis Sci*, **38**, 426–435.

Wilson R., Walker A., Dueker D.K. and Pitts-Crick R. (1982) Risk factors for rate of progression of glaucomatous visual field loss. *Arch Ophthalmol*, **100**, 737–741.

8 Screening for visual field loss

INTRODUCTION
Definition of screening
What does the term screening actually mean? Not surprisingly, it means different things to different people and it is important at the onset of this chapter to clarify its meaning with respect to the eye-caring professions.

If you look in any dictionary, screening will be defined as simply the examination of a large number of individuals to disclose certain characteristics, or a certain disease, such as tuberculosis. Screening tests sort out apparently well persons who probably have a disease from those who probably do not. In this sense screening usually involves the setting up of special centres within the community to which people are invited to come for one or more tests.

Many clinicians now include in their definition of screening the administration of certain additional diagnostic tests to patients already seeking care, such as a blood pressure test to patients consulting their doctor for reasons unconnected with abnormal blood pressure. In this instance, it is only those patients seeking care who benefit from the screening procedures. Some have argued that in these instances the doctor is not screening but case detecting.

So broadly speaking, there are two types of screening programme. In the mass screening programme people are invited along solely for the purpose of being screened. In a practice-based screening programme, screening is applied to patients already seeking care for some unrelated problem.

Both types of screening programme have been conducted by the eye-caring professions. Tuck and Crick (1998) summarize the results from a large number of population-based screening programmes designed to detect glaucoma and there is widespread glaucoma screening of patients seeking routine ophthalmic care.

The requirements of a mass screening programme and a practice-based programme are very different. In a mass screening programme speed of test and high specificity would normally have a higher priority than they would have in a practice-based programme. In any discussion or evaluation of screening programmes it is, therefore, very important to bear in mind the designer's objectives. What might appear an insensitive test for use in a practice-based programme may, for other reasons, be ideal for a mass screening programme.

The role of screening in the detection of glaucoma

In this chapter on screening of the visual field, a great deal of emphasis will be placed upon the detection of the visual field defects associated with primary open angle glaucoma. There are several reasons for this:

(a) **The prevalence of glaucoma**. Glaucoma has a relatively high prevalence for an eye disease, existing in approximately 1.2% of the population over the age of 40 (Tuck and Crick, 1998). The benefits and costs of any screening programme are closely associated with the prevalence of the condition. If the condition we are screening for has a prevalence of 1% and we have a perfect means of discriminating between patients with and without the condition then, on average, we will have to screen 100 patients for every case detected. The benefits of detecting each case must, therefore, be greater than the costs of screening 100 patients. If the condition were to have a prevalence of 0.1% then the benefits must be greater than the costs of screening 1000 patients.

(b) **Significant cause of blindness**. A second reason for concentrating on open angle glaucoma is that it is currently the second largest cause of blindness in most Western nations and as such is a considerable cause of disability and hardship.

(c) **Asymptomatic**. A third reason for concentrating on open angle glaucoma is that in its early stages the condition is asymptomatic and can only be detected by assiduous screening. Many of the other conditions that give rise to visual field loss also give rise to visual symptoms, which will result in the patient seeking medical attention. By the time open angle glaucoma gives rise to visual symptoms the extent of field loss is often severe.

(d) **Discriminatory power**. A fourth reason for concentrating on this condition is that the discriminatory power of a visual field screening test is much higher than that of other glaucoma screening tests (intra-ocular pressure and disc evaluation) (Hill, 1990; Klein *et al.*, 1992). It should be added, however, that the discriminatory power of a combination of tests is much greater than any single test and that, ideally, any screening programme should involve a series of tests.

The remainder of this chapter is going to look at the design of visual field screening tests. It is, however, important to realize that, while visual field tests are better than an evaluation of the optic nerve head or a measure of the IOP, test batteries (e.g. disc evaluation, IOP and visual fields) give superior screening performance to isolated tests (see Harper and Reeves, 1999).

THE DESIGN OF VISUAL FIELD SCREENING TESTS

When designing a screening programme, be it for mass screening or for case detecting in a professional practice, there are a number of questions that need to be answered:

1. What strategy should be used?
2. What areas of the visual field should be investigated?
3. How many locations should be tested?
4. What criteria should be set for passing/failing the test?

Screening strategies

In visual field screening, we are interested in detecting rather than quantifying the extent of any defect. To this end there is almost universal agreement that suprathreshold static strategies are the most appropriate (Heijl, 1976; Greve and Verduin, 1977; Greve, 1979; Dyster-Aas *et al.*, 1980; Kosoko *et al.*, 1983).

These techniques combine a high sensitivity to glaucomatous visual field defects with a short examination time.

Having said that, it is important to emphasize that the comparison of different strategies is fraught with difficulty. While the literature abounds with comparisons of one instrument/strategy versus another, it is very rare for researchers to equate factors such as examination time. It is not unusual for comparisons of sensitivity to be made between full threshold tests, which take 15 minutes to perform, and suprathreshold tests that take less than 5 minutes to perform. Comparisons are made even more difficult by the fact that there are many different types of kinetic, threshold and suprathreshold tests (see Chapter 3).

Even after taking into account all the problems, the consensus of opinion remains that static suprathreshold strategies are best for screening/detecting early loss. It can also be stated, on an empirical basis, that eccentrically compensated strategies (those in which the intensity of the suprathreshold stimulus increases towards the peripheral regions of the field to compensate for the normal reduction in sensitivity with eccentricity) will be superior to strategies which present the stimuli at a constant intensity across the whole visual field.

Another aspect of suprathreshold tests that it is important to take into account is the way in which they establish the suprathreshold test intensity. Some suprathreshold strategies simply set the intensity at a fixed level for all patients (fixed intensity suprathreshold test) (Harrington and Flocks, 1959); others adjust the test intensity according to the age of the patient (age-related suprathreshold test) (Bedwell, 1982); while still others set the test intensity according to an estimate of the patient's threshold made at the beginning of the examination (threshold-related suprathreshold test). While it is clear that the more sophisticated threshold-related test strategy will produce more accurate results (less errors) this is only achieved at the expense of increased testing time.

Let us investigate this last point a little more closely. If for the moment we consider that the practitioner has a fixed time in which to examine the visual field, should that practitoner choose, for example, an age-related strategy or a threshold-related one? In the first instance, because there is no time spent on establishing the threshold, an increased amount of time will be available for testing the visual field, i.e. it will be

possible to test more locations. In the second instance, establishing the threshold on each patient will result in more accurate results and fewer errors. But do the benefits of the increased accuracy of a threshold-related test outweigh the disadvantages of presenting less stimuli? Unfortunately, there is no simple answer to this question. There are, however, two factors that should be taken into account when trying to answer it!

(a) **The amount of time available**. As will be shown in a later section of this chapter, there is a logarithmic relationship between the sensitivity of a test and the number of test locations (see Figure 8.2). Increasing the number of stimuli has a much more significant effect upon sensitivity when the initial number of test locations is small than it does when the number is large. In other words, any benefits of an age-related strategy are more likely to be evident when the number of test locations is small.

(b) **The time taken to train the patient at the beginning of the examination**. All strategies require some training and it is often possible to combine training with establishing the threshold in a threshold-related strategy. In this instance the overall time saved in using an age-related strategy may be small.

After taking all these factors into account, most clinicians involved in practice-based screening have concluded that the advantages of a threshold-related test outweigh those of an age-related test.

Another aspect to be considered when deciding upon the appropriate strategy is whether it is better to use single or multiple stimulus presentations. With a multiple stimulus strategy, the perimetrist presents patterns of, usually, 2, 3 or 4 stimuli and the patient verbally reports how many they see. The multiple stimulus technique is much faster than a single stimulus one, taking only half the time to present the same number of stimuli (Henson and Anderson, 1989) (see Chapter 3 for more details concerning the advantages and disadvantages of multiple stimulus techniques). In a screening environment this time advantage is of very real significance.

Several researchers have proposed using a combination of both static and kinetic strategies to screen the visual field (Rock *et al.*, 1973; Miller *et al.*, 1989). The relative merits of these strategies are hard to evaluate as many of the current generation of perimeters cannot present kinetic stimuli. Again, it should be stressed that it is not simply a matter of looking at how many additional defects will be found by including a kinetic element. The clinician has to consider what benefits might accrue from spending the same amount of additional time on alternative forms of testing.

So where does this leave us with respect to choosing a strategy for screening? When screening is performed as an additional test to patients already consulting a professional, the majority of practitioners have opted to use a threshold-related suprathreshold test with either single or multiple stimuli. The majority of mass screening programmes have also chosen to use threshold-related suprathreshold strategies.

POSITION OF STIMULI

Where should the stimuli be placed? Should they be concentrated in those regions of the field where most defects are known to occur or should they be evenly distributed? Should they be confined to the central region of the field or should they include the periphery?

Area to be covered

The visual field has historically always been divided into two sections, the central field extending out to approximately 30 degrees of eccentricity, and the peripheral field extending from 30 degrees to the absolute edge of the field (sea of blindness). Currently, the vast majority of screening strategies confine themselves to the central field. There are two reasons for this:

(i) It is in this region that most defects first appear (particularly in glaucoma).

(ii) It is the region which is functionally more important.

A number of research papers have investigated the effects of ignoring the peripheral field (LeBlanc and Becker, 1971; Werner and Beroskow, 1979; LeBlanc *et al.*, 1985; Stewart *et al.*, 1988; Miller *et al.*, 1989; Stewart and Schields, 1991). They report that anywhere between 1 and 15% of patients with glaucomatous field loss have defects that lie solely outside the central 30 degrees. The reported incidence of these defects is inversely proportional to the quality of both central and peripheral examinations. The more carefully one examines the central

field, the less often isolated peripheral defects are found. Again, this leaves the clinician questioning whether any time spent on screening the peripheral field could not have been just as well spent on examining the central field more thoroughly. This is especially true when consideration is given to the problems encountered with artefacts due to the correcting lens and eyelid, which primarily occur outside the central 25 degrees (for further details of parameters that affect the visual field see Chapter 5).

Distribution of stimuli

The distribution of stimuli within a screening programme varies considerably from one screening strategy to another. They can be placed on a square matrix, a radial matrix, an annular matrix (see Figure 8.1), or in relation to the frequency distribution of glaucomatous defects. Henson *et al.*, (1988) demonstrated that improved sensitivities could be obtained if the stimuli were distributed in proportion to the frequency distribution of glaucoma defects. This advantage, however, disappears when the number of test locations becomes large (greater than 30). This is due to the large variability in the location of glaucomatous defects. While it is true to say that glaucomatous defects most frequently occur at certain test locations (see Chapter 7), they can occur almost anywhere. Thus, as the number of test locations increases, a point is reached where the frequency of undetected defects, in any given sample, is the same for both high and low risk areas. At this point the increased likelihood of detecting additional defects is the same no matter where the additional stimuli are placed.

NUMBER OF STIMULI

How many test locations do we need in a screening programme? If only a few locations are tested obviously there is a danger of defects going undetected. On the other hand, as the number of test locations increases so too does the testing time.

The relationship between the number of test locations and the sensitivity of a screening strategy was derived by Henson *et al.*, (1988) and Johnson and Keltner (1988). It was found to be logarithmic: as the number of test locations increased, so too did the test sensitivity (see Figure 8.2).

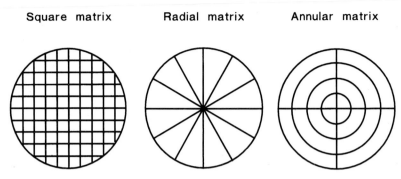

Fig. 8.1   *Different matrices used in the distribution of stimuli.*

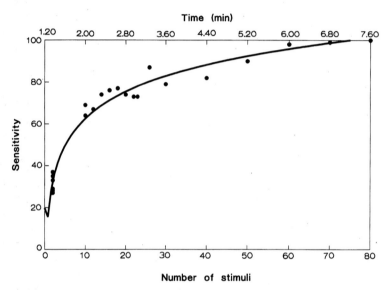

Fig. 8.2   *The relationship between the number of test locations and the sensitivity of a screening test. Also given is the time taken to examine both eyes with a multiple stimulus, threshold-related suprathreshold test.*

An interesting finding to come out of this research was the relatively high sensitivities reached with relatively few stimuli; 80% sensitivity with only 30 stimuli – the criteria for failing the test being set at missing one or more, non-blind spot, stimuli.

In Figure 8.2 the abscissa also gives the testing time for a multiple stimulus suprathreshold test. For single stimulus suprathreshold tests you need to double the testing time (these times are based upon examinations of patients without visual field loss).

Unfortunately, there is no simple answer to the question of how many test locations should be included within a screening strategy. Looking at the current generation of instruments there also seems to be little consensus of opinion. Some strategies test only a dozen or so locations while others test 60 or more. The Henson range of perimeters rather than opt for a fixed number of test locations within a screening strategy have adopted what they call a graded approach to screening. The screening test starts off with just 26 test locations and strict pass/fail criteria (one missed stimulus outside of the blind spot region). This combines a relatively high sensitivity with a low specificity (approximately 80%; Harper and Reeves; 1999) and a very short examination time (less than 5 minutes for both eyes). Any patient who fails this test is then subjected to further testing (the number of test stimuli increasing to 68 and then 136) in order to improve the test specificity. This strategy has been evaluated by Sponsel *et al.*, (1995), who reported that it had a sensitivity of 84% and a specificity of 100%. The sensitivity increased to 97% for cases of moderate to advanced visual field loss.

A recent proposal has been that the number of stimuli tested should be based upon the prior probability of the patient having glaucoma. For example, an 80-year-old with a family history of glaucoma has a higher probability of having glaucoma than a 40-year-old with no family history of glaucoma. Put another way, the perimetrist should continue to present stimuli until he or she reaches a certain confidence level for either the presence, or absence, of a visual field defect.

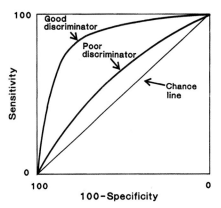

Fig. 8.3 *Example of two ROC curves.*

PASS/FAIL CRITERIA

The terms sensitivity and specificity are widely used both within this text and within the literature to describe the merits or failings of any particular instrument/strategy. Like all statistical measures, they are often misused and even more widely misunderstood. Before describing the problems and misconceptions that often arise when using these terms let us attempt a definition. Sensitivity is the percentage of patients who both (a) have the condition and (b) who fail the test.

$$\text{Sensitivity} = \frac{\text{Number of defectives failing} \times 100}{\text{Total number of defectives}}$$

(Sensitivity is also known as the true positive rate, hit rate or probability of detection).

Specificity is the percentage of patients who both (a) do not have the condition and (b) pass the test.

$$\text{Specificity} = \frac{\text{Number of normals passing} \times 100}{\text{Number of normals tested}}$$

(Specificity is also known as the true negative rate or correct rejection rate).

While measures of sensitivity and specificity are very valuable in that they give an estimate of the worth of any particular test, they are dependent upon the pass/fail criteria used. If the criteria are altered so that it becomes more difficult for a normal patient to fail the test then two things happen: (a) the test becomes more specific and (b) it becomes less sensitive. The interdependence of sensitivity and specificity and their relationship with the pass/fail criteria has made it very difficult to compare one

strategy with another. For example, which is the better strategy, one that has a sensitivity of 90% and a specificity of 70% or one that has a sensitivity of 70% and a specificity of 90%?

Fortunately, there are ways of overcoming these problems. Massof and Emmel (1987) have described techniques of assessing tests that are criterion free. They are based upon the construction of an ROC (relative operating characteristic) curve which is a plot of sensitivity on the ordinate versus false positive rate on the abscissa (100% minus specificity) for a whole series of different pass/fail criteria. Figure 8.3 represents a typical ROC curve. Each point on the curve represents the sensitivity and specificity of a unique set of criteria. The curve is a demonstration of how sensitivity and specificity co-vary with criteria. The diagonal line represents chance performance where sensitivity and specificity are equal. When a result falls on this line, the test, allied with the specific set of criteria is unable to differentiate between patients who do and those who do not have the condition, i.e. it is useless.

Different tests, allied with their different sets of criteria, will give different ROC curves. Tests which are poor at discriminating between normals and defectives will give ROC curves which are close to the chance line. Those that are good at discriminating between these two populations will approach the upper left-hand corner, which corresponds to 100% sensitive and 100% specific.

If we were looking for a criterion-free index of a test's performance, then the area underneath the ROC curve would seem to fit the bill. An ROC curve that follows the chance line will have an area of 0.5, while one that follows the ordinate to the top left hand corner and then proceeds along the top edge will have an area of 1. A test whose area underneath its ROC curve is 1 is a perfect discriminator between normals and defectives, there being no false positives or false negatives. Tests can, therefore, be evaluated by simply measuring the area under their ROC curve. The greater the area, the better the test is at discriminating between normal and defective patients.*

A point worth mentioning here, for those who want to get more involved in this subject, is that this type of measure becomes less valuable at discriminating between tests when the area under the ROC curve approaches unity. A significant increase in test performance, say from 98 to 99% specificity – a 50% reduction in the number of false positives – will have a relatively insignificant effect upon the area under the ROC curve.

Selection of optimal pass/fail criteria

ROC curves can also be used to select the optimal pass/fail criteria. In selecting these, attention has to be given to the costs and benefits of false positive and false negative test outcomes.

Costs of a false positive outcome

In an optometric or ophthalmological environment, the costs of a false positive may be very low as anybody who fails the visual field screening test can easily be subjected to additional tests. These would, hopefully, reduce the number of patients falsely referred by optometrists or falsely treated by ophthalmologists to a very low level. In a mass screening situation, the cost of a false positive could be much higher as the patient, after failing the test, would be referred to a professional for further examination, thereby incurring a great deal of extra expense.

Costs of a false negative outcome

The costs of a false negative are dependent upon a whole series of factors such as likely prognosis, costs of treatment etc. The reader interested in delving

further into this topic is recommended to read the following papers: Eddy *et al.*, (1983), Keltner and Johnson (1983), Levi and Schwartz (1983), Gottlieb *et al.*, (1983).

An important factor relating to false positive test outcomes, which is not covered in the above references, is the severity of the defect. Most clinicians would view the failure to detect an advanced field defect as more serious than the failure to detect subtle, early loss. Quantifying this is, however, fraught with difficulty and most evaluations of screening strategies view the failure to detect any defect as equal, which is clearly not the case.

In establishing optimal pass/fail criteria, attention also has to be given to the probabilities of any given condition being present or absent. As the condition becomes increasingly rare so the optimal criteria (those that produce the minimum number of errors weighted for benefits and costs) shift towards higher specificity. This effect is diagrammatically represented in Figure 8.4. When looking at this diagram, the reader should bear in mind that the incidence of field defects in an optometric practice is likely to be in the order of 2%, while the incidence in a referred population may be as high as 50%.

All these factors can be put together in the form of an equation which gives the slope of the tangent to the ROC curve at the point of optimal criteria (Hill, 1987).

$$\text{Slope} = \frac{p(D-) \times (\text{Benefit TN} + \text{Cost FP})}{p(D+) \times (\text{Benefit TP} + \text{Cost FN})}$$

where P(D+) and P(D−) are the probabilities of a field defect being present and TN, TP, FP and FN represent True Negative, True Positive, False Positive and False Negative respectively.

By way of illustration, consider the following two examples. In the first, the costs and benefits are worked out to give a slope of 1, while, in the second they produce a slope of 0.25. Figure 8.5 gives a hypothetical ROC curve where each point on the curve represents a specific set of pass/fail criteria. Two lines, one with a slope of 1 and the other with a slope of 0.25, have been drawn to form a tangent with the ROC curve. The point at which they touch the curve represents the optimal set of criteria for the two sets of conditions.

Using ROC curves to derive both a criteria-free estimate of a test's performance and optimal pass/fail

---

* In this instance, ROC curves have been advocated for use in comparing one test/strategy with another and to look at optimal pass/fail criteria. They can also be used in many other ways. For example they can be used to compare different suprathreshold test increments, different numbers of test stimuli or any other factor whose parameters can affect sensitivity and specificity.

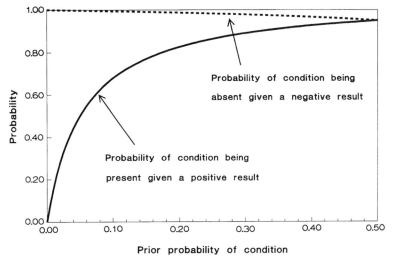

Fig. 8.4 *Relationship between the prior probability of a condition and the probability of the condition being present or absent given a positive or negative test result.*

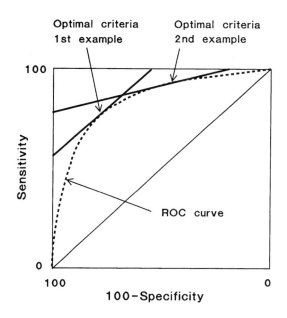

Fig. 8.5 *Use of ROC curve to establish optimal criteria.*

criteria is still in its infancy. The majority of clinical papers still compare one test with another by looking at individual measures of sensitivity and specificity for a unique, but often arbitrary, set of criteria. It is hoped that the elegance of ROC analysis will in the future lead to more thorough test evaluations and more care in selecting pass/fail criteria.

REFERENCES

Bedwell C.H. (1982) *Visual Fields. A Basis for Efficient Investigation*, Butterworths, London.

Dyster-Aas K., Heijl A. and Lundquist L. (1980) Computerised visual field screening in the management of patients with ocular hypertension. *Acta Ophthalmol*, **58**, 918–928.

Eddy D.M., Sanders L.E. and Eddy J.F. (1983) The value of screening for glaucoma with tonometry. *Surv Ophthalmol*, **28**, 194–205.

Gottlieb L.K., Schwartz B. and Pauker S.G. (1983) Glaucoma screening. A cost-effective analysis. *Surv Ophthalmol*, **28**, 206–226.

Greve E.L. (1979) Some aspects of visual field examination related to strategies for detection and assessment phase. *Doc Ophthalmol Proc Series*, **22**, 15–28.

Greve E.L. and Verduin W.M. (1977) Detection of early glaucomatous damage, part 1. Visual field examination. *Doc Ophthalmol Proc Series*, **14**, 103–114.

Harper R.A. and Reeves B.C. (1999) Glaucoma screening: the importance of combining test data. *Optom Vis Sci*, **76**, 537–543.

Harrington D.O. and Flocks M. (1959) The multiple-pattern method of visual field examination. A five year evaluation of its effectiveness as a screening technique. *Arch Ophthalmol*, **61**, 755–765.

Henson D.B. and Anderson R. (1989) Thresholds using single and multiple stimulus presentations. In *Perimetry Update 1988/1989* (ed. Heijl A.). Kugler & Ghedini, Amsterdam, pp. 191–196.

Henson D.B., Chauhan B.C. and Hobley A. (1988) Screening for glaucomatous visual field defects: the relationship between sensitivity, specificity and the number of test locations. *Ophthal Physiol Opt*, **8**, 123–127.

Heijl A. (1976) Automatic perimetry in glaucoma visual field screening: a clinical study. *Graefe Arch Clin Exp Ophthalmol*, **200**, 21–37.

Hill A.R. (1987) Making decisions in ophthalmology. In *Retinal Research* Volume 6 (eds Osborne N.N. and Chader G.J.). Pergamon, Oxford, pp. 207–244.

Hill A.R. (1990) *Primary Open-Angle Glaucoma and Its Detection*. British College of Optometrists.

Johnson C.A. and Keltner J.L. (1988) Computer analysis of visual field loss and optimization of automated perimetric test strategies. *Ophthalmol*, **88**, 1058–1065.

Keltner J.L. and Johnson C.A. (1983) Screening for visual field abnormalities with automated perimetry. *Surv Ophthalmol*, **28**, 175–183.

Klein B.E.K., Klein R., Sponsel W.E., Franke T., Cantor L.B., Martone J. *et al.* (1992) Prevalence of glaucoma. The Beaver Dam eye study. *Ophthalmology*, **99**, 1499–1504.

Kosoko O., Sommer A. and Auer C. (1983) Screening with automated perimetry using a threshold related three-level algorithm. *Ophthalmol*, **93**, 882–886.

LeBlanc R.P. and Becker B. (1971) Peripheral nasal field defects in glaucoma. *Am J Ophthalmol*, **72**, 415–419.

LeBlanc R.P., Lee A. and Baxter M. (1985) Peripheral nasal field defects. *Doc Ophthalmol Proc Series*, **42**, 377–381.

Levi L. and Schwartz B. (1983) Glaucoma screening in the health care setting. *Surv Ophthalmol*, **28**, 164–174.

Massof R.W. and Emmel T.C. (1987) Criterion-free parameter-free distribution-independent index of diagnostic test performance. *Appl Opt*, **26**, 1395–1408.

Miller K.N., Shields M.B. and Ollie A.R. (1989) Automated kinetic perimetry with two peripheral isopters in glaucoma. *Arch Ophthalmol*, **107**, 1316–1320.

Rabin S., Kolesar P., Podos S.M. and Wilensky J.T. (1981) A visual field screening protocol for glaucoma. *Am J Ophthalmol*, **92**, 530–535.

Rock W.J., Drance S.M. and Morgan R.W. (1973) Visual field screening in glaucoma. *Arch Ophthalmol*, **89**, 287–290.

Sponsel W.E., Ritch R., Stamper R., Higginbotham E.J., Anderson D.R., Wilson M.R. and Zimmerman T.J. (1995) Prevent Blindness America visual field screening study. *Am J Ophthalmol*, **120**, 699–708.

Stewart W.C. and Schields M.B. (1991) The peripheral visual field in glaucoma: Re-evaluation in the age of automated perimetry. *Surv Ophthalmol*, **36**, 59–69.

Stewart W.C., Schields M.B. and Ollie A.R. (1988) Peripheral visual fields testing by automated kinetic perimetry in glaucoma. *Arch Ophthalmol*, **106**, 202–206.

Tuck M.W. and Crick R.P. (1998) The age distribution of primary open angle glaucoma. *Ophthalmic Epidemiol*, **5**, 173–183.

Werner E.B. and Beraskow J. (1979) Peripheral nasal field defects in glaucoma. *Ophthalmol*, **86**, 1875–1888.

9 Quantification of visual field data

INTRODUCTION AND THE VALUE OF QUANTIFICATION

Visual field data is normally presented in a graphical format for interpretation by the clinician, i.e. a visual field chart. The term quantification refers to the reduction of the data presented in the field chart to either one or a series of different numbers that represent certain characteristics of the visual field data. The numbers may represent the extent of field loss or the variability in the patient's responses. The results of any quantification are normally included on the visual field chart (see Figure 9.1).

Now to some readers the provision of these numbers may initially appear as an over-complicated waste of time. You can look at a field chart and see whether a defect exists and whether it has changed so why get involved in lots of complicated mathematics to state the obvious? Well, there are three important situations where the quantification of results is of value.

Monitoring progressive loss

The number(s) derived from the quantification system can be used to monitor a patient's visual field. In conditions such as glaucoma, where there may be progressive visual field loss, the different quantification scores allow us to derive an estimate of the rate of field loss. Different forms of therapy can then be tried to see what effect they have upon the rate of loss. Quantification is of particular value when a clinician wishes to conduct a clinical trial involving a large number of patients. It might well be argued that simple visual inspection of the field charts could provide the clinician with a very good estimate of what is

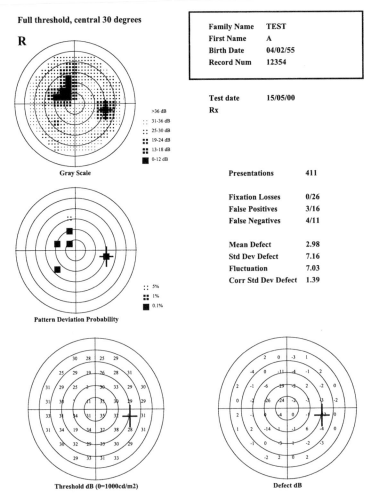

Fig. 9.1 *Example of a field chart in which the global indices 'Mean Defect', 'Std Dev Defect', 'Fluctuation' and 'Corr Std Dev Defect' are given.*

happening. However, this is not the case when the clinician is presented with 100 sets of visual field records in which 50 have been using one form of medication while the other 50 have been using another. To obtain a reliable estimate of which is the better form of treatment it is now essential to have some form of quantification.

Detecting field loss

Quantification can be of value in assessing whether a significant defect exists. By comparing the patient's quantified result with those from a normal population the perimetrist, or perimeter, can compute the like-

lihood of the patient's visual field being normal. For example, the perimetrist may conclude that there is less than a 1 in 1000 chance that the current field result has come from a patient with a normal visual field.

Measuring the extent of loss

The number(s) derived from the quantification system can be used to estimate how much of the visual field has been lost. This is particularly important in litigation cases where a patient is claiming damages for visual loss or impairment. With the aid of an accepted quantification system an ophthalmologist can report to the court that the patient has lost a given percentage of their visual field.

The need for different forms of quantification

The three situations described above are very different and a quantification system developed for one situation will not necessarily be suitable for the other two. It could be argued that instruments should incorporate several different quantification systems, one for detecting field loss, one for monitoring field loss and one for giving an estimate of functional loss.

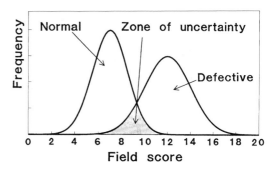

Fig. 9.2 *Two hypothetical distributions. One from a normal population and one from a defective population. The overlap area represents a zone of uncertainty where a patient may be from either population.*

VARIABILITY

Before going on to describe some of the commonly used quantification systems, it is important to first point out that the results of any visual field examination are subject to a certain amount of variability. In a system that quantifies the visual field this variability is represented by changes in the numerical values which represent the visual field.

Where a quantification system is being used to monitor loss it is important to assess the amount of variability in the results. It is not simply a matter of whether the numerical values have changed since the last field test, but rather whether they have changed by a significant amount. Since such statements can only be made if we know how much variability to expect, any quantification system must include estimates of the normal range of values so that the clinician can then establish the significance of the result.

This problem is particularly acute in glaucoma where there is an increase in the variability of the results beyond that seen in normal patients (see Chapter 2, p. 20). In such instances it is often necessary to have several measures of the field before a decision can be made on whether or not the visual field defect is progressing.

Similarly, when a quantification system is being used to assess whether or not a patient has a visual field defect (establishing loss), the variability between normals means that it is not so much a question as to whether they do or do not have a defect but rather one of whether their results are significantly different from the norm. Once again, to make such statements it is essential that we know what the normal range of values is.

EVALUATING QUANTIFICATION SYSTEMS

A very important factor in the evaluation of any quantification system is the definition of the condition one is trying to detect. It is often very difficult to get a universally accepted definition: for example, how do we define a glaucomatous eye? If the definition is changed then this can have a very significant effect upon the apparent accuracy of the quantification system.

One way of assessing the merits of a quantification system is to look at the distribution of results from both normal and defective populations. Figure 9.2 gives hypothetical results from a quantification system designed to detect glaucoma. We can see from this figure that normal subjects have a mean value of 7 with a standard deviation (due to inherent variability) of 1.5 and that the defective population has a mean value of 12 with a standard deviation of 3. On average we can say that this quantification system works because those with glaucoma have higher scores than those without. There is, however, a zone of uncertainty between scores of 6 and 12 at which significant numbers of both normal and glaucomatous patients lie. With field scores that fall within this range we cannot say with any degree of confidence that a patient does or does not have a defect.

Figure 9.3 gives the results from a different hypothetical quantification system. In this instance the range of normal values is much smaller (mean 3, standard deviation 1), while the range of glaucoma values is similar to that of the previous quantification system. The zone of uncertainty has almost totally disappeared and we could rightly conclude that this

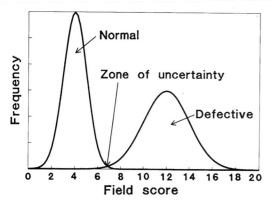

Fig. 9.3 *Two more hypothetical populations in which there is practically no zone of uncertainty.*

quantification system is better than the previous one at differentiating between normal and glaucomatous eyes.

This example has been based upon a quantification system designed to differentiate between normal and glaucomatous eyes. Similar arguments apply to systems designed to monitor glaucomatous loss, only in this case the two populations would be of glaucomats with and without progressive loss rather than normal and glaucomatous eyes.

Comparing quantification systems

Strictly speaking, one quantification system can only be compared with another when they are both applied to the same group of patients. Differences in the type of field loss included in the patient group can have significant effects upon the apparent accuracy of the quantification system.

Suppose, for example, we had two groups of patients. The first group contains patients who are either normal or who have advanced visual field loss, while the second group contains patients who are either normal or have subtle early visual field loss. If the quantification system is applied to the first group then it would more than likely come up with a clear segregation of normals from defectives. The same quantification system applied to the second group would yield much more ambiguous results. The difference is due to the differences in the composition of the two groups and not to the quantification system. Hence, for those wishing to evaluate different quantification systems it is important to do so on the same group of patients, or at least on very carefully matched

groups of patients. As you can imagine this puts very severe limitations on our ability to assess different systems. One novel approach to this problem, which has to date seen little use, is to evaluate quantification techniques on a computer model simulating both normal and defective eyes (Shapiro *et al.*, 1989).

THE DEVELOPMENT OF QUANTIFICATION SYSTEMS

Some of the quantification systems to be described below are very basic while others are highly complex. Each system seems to have its own natural evolution. It starts off as a simple idea involving elementary mathematical calculations. It is then found to have certain limitations that can be corrected for by the addition of more parameters to the calculation, (i.e. by increasing its complexity). This new system is then found to have yet other limitations that were not recognized earlier on; these are again corrected for by more complex calculations. This process continues until the equations become so complex that very few people understand exactly how the result is obtained. There is an inherent danger here that users who do not appreciate how the values are calculated will not understand the limitations of the system. There is a strong case, therefore, for keeping quantification systems as simple as possible and thereby ensuring that any limitations are understood by its users.

TYPES OF QUANTIFICATION SYSTEM

There are literally hundreds of ways in which visual field results can be quantified and the rest of this chapter will cover those techniques that have reached a certain amount of acceptability. This may have resulted from the techniques being (a) recommended by organizations such as the American Medical Association, (b) incorporated into instruments which have reached a certain popularity or (c) simply novel.

The techniques are broadly divided into the following categories:

1. those that apply to the kinetic technique of examination;
2. those that apply to suprathreshold static techniques of examination;
3. those that apply to static threshold techniques;
4. novel techniques.

Quantifying the results from kinetic perimetry

Before getting involved in the details of the various kinetic quantification systems it is possibly worth pointing out that kinetic techniques and quantification systems have never been very good bedfellows.

In part, this might be due to the lack of any widely used commercial package, although I suspect that the real reason is the lack of control over many of the parameters, such as speed of stimulus movement, which affect the results. In an ideal world quantification systems should be independent of the operator.

Area measurements from isopter diagrams

One of the simplest ways of quantifying the results from a kinetic visual field examination is to measure the area enclosed by a given isopter on the visual field chart. This measurement can then be compared to a set of normal values, or monitored over a period of time to see if there is any deterioration or improvement.

By changing the stimulus strength, and hence the area covered by the isopter, this technique can be used to monitor the whole of the visual field or just the central region.

In practice, visual field charts are normally placed on a digitizing tablet or a planimeter from which the area enclosed by an isopter is automatically calculated (Hart and Hartz, 1981; Pe'er *et al.*, 1983).

A major benefit of this technique is that it can be used retrospectively, i.e. to analyse data that has already been collected. In the majority of clinics there are visual field records dating back many years and to be able to retrospectively analyse this data is of obvious value. Another advantage of this technique is its simplicity. It is easily understood and the limitations (these are discussed below) readily appreciated.

A major shortcoming of the technique is its insensitivity to small central scotomas and over-sensitivity to slight contractions of the peripheral field. It gives even weighting to all regions of the field and does not acknowledge that the central field is functionally more important. Figures 9.4 and 9.5 give two examples. In the first, there is a slight contraction of the peripheral field that could very well be caused by a prominent nose, while in the second there is a paracentral scotoma. When quantified with an area measuring technique both charts give the same result!

This limitation can be partially overcome by altering the visual field projection; giving the central

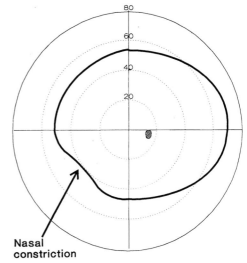

Nasal constriction

Fig. 9.4 *Isopter diagram showing an area of nasal constriction, which could easily be due to a prominent nose.*

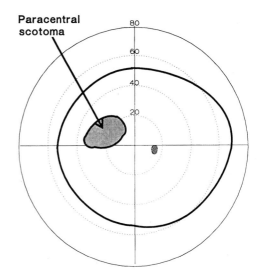

Paracentral scotoma

Fig. 9.5 *Isopter diagram showing a paracentral scotoma.*

region more dominance than the periphery. There are two ways in which this can be achieved.

(i) The instrument used to collect the data could be adjusted such that the central field represented a larger area on the chart.

(ii) The digitiser, or planimeter, could be adjusted to give increased weighting to the central field.

The latter technique is more attractive because it still allows the clinician to analyse data retrospectively and, via software changes, to use different projections. There are, however, disadvantages to altering the projection. First, projections other than those currently used in the Goldmann instrument have not found wide acceptance and, second, such systems are more complex and, as a consequence, not so easily understood. In addition no modification to the projection will enable an area measuring technique to differentiate between central scotoma and peripheral contractions.

Finally, there is the additional problem of finding a projection for which there is general acceptance amongst the eye-caring professions.

Area measuring techniques can be used with different isopters to give a volumetric measure of field loss. This modification was used by Mikelberg *et al.*, (1986) and Schultzer *et al.*, (1987) to report on both the rate of progression of glaucomatous loss in the central field and on the relative importance of the central and peripheral field in monitoring progression.

Area measurements with Esterman grids
Esterman (1982, 1985) describes a modification to the area measuring technique in which the visual field is weighted according to its functional importance. The technique is very simple and does not require vast amounts of investment in computer technology. The clinician simply places an overlay on top of a field chart. On the overlay there is a grid of rectangles, the size of which varies across the field (see Figure 9.6). By simply counting the number of spots falling within a given isopter, there being one in each rectangle, the clinician obtains a percentage score of the functional field. Overlays have been generated for

the central field as measured with a tangent screen (Esterman, 1967), the peripheral field (Esterman, 1968) and the binocular field (Esterman, 1982).

Esterman's scoring system was adopted in 1984 by the American Medical Association as a method of measuring visual disability and has, therefore, been widely used for litigation purposes. The technique was never intended to be used for either the detection or the monitoring of visual field loss. The binocular version is, however, widely used in the UK as a driver's test. It is not necessary for drivers to see all the Esterman test points but sufficient to meet the UK's current driving standard.

The size and location of the rectangles used in the Esterman system were derived after careful assessment of how well patients with established visual field loss performed. They are not based upon any known projection of the visual field.

Radial summation
The radial summation technique is used to quantify the extent of field plotted with isopter diagrams. Its origins date back to 1958 when the American Medical Association first devised a system to quantify the extent of field loss. The field was first plotted with a 3/330 white target and then the extent of the field along eight different meridians was measured and the values added together (see Figure 9.7). The radial sum of a normal field was approximately 500 and a percentage of the normal score could be obtained by simply dividing the sum by 5.

The attractions of this technique are again its simplicity and the fact that it does not rely upon the

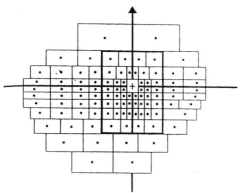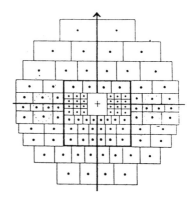

Fig. 9.6 *Esterman grid for the whole field and for central 30 degrees.*

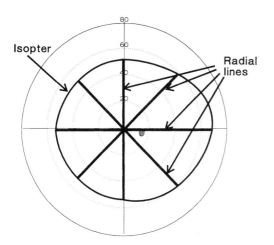

Fig. 9.7 *Eight radial lines used in the radial summation technique which was adopted by the American Medical Association.*

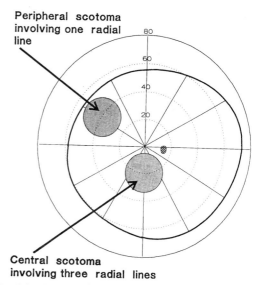

Fig. 9.8 *Diagram demonstrating how the effect upon the summation score will be influenced by the position of a scotoma.*

existence of sophisticated instrumentation for either the collection of the data or the analysis of the results. Its disadvantages are that fairly large central defects can exist without having any significant effect upon the overall score and that it is insensitive to small changes in the visual field unless they occur in a radial direction.

A variation of this technique was used by Smith (1968) to evaluate the central 40 degrees of the visual field. Smith (1968) used a total of 24 radial lines (one every 15 degrees) on a Goldmann perimeter and summed the results out to 40 degrees. The maximum score (960) was then divided by 9.6 to give a percentage score of the residual central field. By using a larger number of radial lines the technique became more sensitive to small central defects at the cost of a slightly increased computation time.

The radial summation technique has been developed even further by Sponsel *et al.* (1984). They entered the Goldmann visual field results into a small microcomputer system with the aid of a digitizing tablet. The computer calculated the sum of 24 radial lines and compared this value to a set of normal data in order to give a percentage score. Sponsel's system could be used with several different Goldmann stimuli in order to obtain estimates of both central and peripheral field losses.

An important point concerning this technique is that by measuring the radial sum we are giving greater importance to the central region of the field.

If we consider a given sized scotoma located in the central field then it will affect a greater number of radial lines than the same sized scotoma located in the peripheral field (see Figure 9.8). The technique is, however, still relatively insensitive to central scotoma and is incapable of differentiating between nasal steps, central scotoma and peripheral contraction.

Kinetic visual field indices
The use of three visual field indices to represent the extent of glaucomatous loss was proposed by Flammer *et al.*, (1985) (see section on quantifying results from full-threshold techniques for more details). An analogous set of indices has been developed for the automated Goldmann bowl perimeter (Perikon) (Capris *et al.*, 1987). These indices, kinetic mean defect, kinetic loss variance, kinetic corrected loss variance and kinetic short-term fluctuation, are calculated with identical formulae to those developed by Flammer *et al.*, (1985) only instead of using sensitivity measures the calculations use isopter eccentricity along 16 different meridians.

Quantifying results from static suprathreshold techniques

Suprathreshold techniques are primarily used to screen for visual field defects and the quantification systems developed for these techniques have largely been designed to differentiate between normals and those with significant visual field loss.

Number of missed stimuli

One of the simplest ways of quantifying the results from either a one-level or a gradient-adapted supra-threshold technique is to count the number of missed stimuli and give the result as a percentage of the total number of stimuli. Such systems, while appearing crude, are remarkably robust and give estimates of field loss that agree well with those of clinical ophthalmologists (Hobley, 1986).

This simple system can be improved by taking account of defect depth, greater importance being given to deeper defects, an improvement which requires the suprathreshold technique to retest missed stimuli at higher intensities.

Cluster analysis

One of the shortcomings of using a simple count of missed stimuli is that it cannot differentiate between a few scattered misses and a cluster of missed stimuli (see Figure 9.9). The former might simply mean that the patient is unreliable while the latter is a very powerful indicator of a defect. Cluster analysis of suprathreshold data has been used by Henson and Dix (1984), Henson et al., (1984) and Chauhan et al., (1990) in an evaluation of results obtained with a Friedmann Visual Field Analyser. They demonstrated that the addition of a clustering routine had a significant effect upon the ability of the quantification system to differentiate between normal patients and those with early glaucomatous loss.

Measuring extent of field loss

While, as pointed out at the beginning of this section, suprathreshold techniques are primarily used to screen for visual field defects, one or two systems have been developed to quantify the extent of field loss. The system developed for the Henson CFS2000/CFA3000 (Henson and Bryson, 1987), gives a measure of the field survival (100% minus field loss). A series of equations, which take into account the number, depth and cluster properties of the missed stimuli, are used to give results which mirror those of a group of experts (see Hobley, 1986).

Quantifying the results from static threshold strategies

Flammer et al., (1985) proposed that the visual field defects associated with glaucoma could be divided into three different categories:

1. Those that cause an overall depression in the sensitivity of the eye.
2. Those that cause local defects.
3. Those that cause an increase in the variability of results.

They also proposed that the visual field records of glaucoma patients and glaucoma suspects should be quantified to give three indices, one for each of the three categories. They called these three indices mean defect, corrected loss variation and short-term fluctuation.

The concept of using three separate indices has found very wide acceptance within the ophthalmological professions and many visual field instruments now incorporate, as part of their software, a set of algorithms which compute these or very similar indices. The name given to these indices varies from one instrument to another, as does the form of calculation (in the Humphrey instrument they are called mean deviation, corrected pattern standard deviation and short-term fluctuation) but the concept behind the indices remains the same, i.e. that they represent the three types of visual field damage seen in glaucoma.

In the following paragraphs, the three indices developed by Flammer et al., (1985) will be described in more detail. There follows a description of the differences between these indices and those incorporated in the Humphrey Visual Field Analyzer. Finally, there are descriptions of some alternative empirical methods of defining when a defect does or does not exist which are based upon parameters such as the number and depth of defects. Several grading systems based upon this type of analysis are also described.

Octopus indices

Mean defect. The mean defect value is designed to give a measure of the overall loss in sensitivity. Each tested location is compared with that from a population of age matched normal values. The results are then averaged to give the mean defect (see Figure 9.10) (Flammer et al., 1985). The mean defect is affected

Multiple stimulus, suprathreshold, central 25 degrees.

Family Name
First Name
Birth Date
Record Num

Test date   12/10/99
RxR
RxL

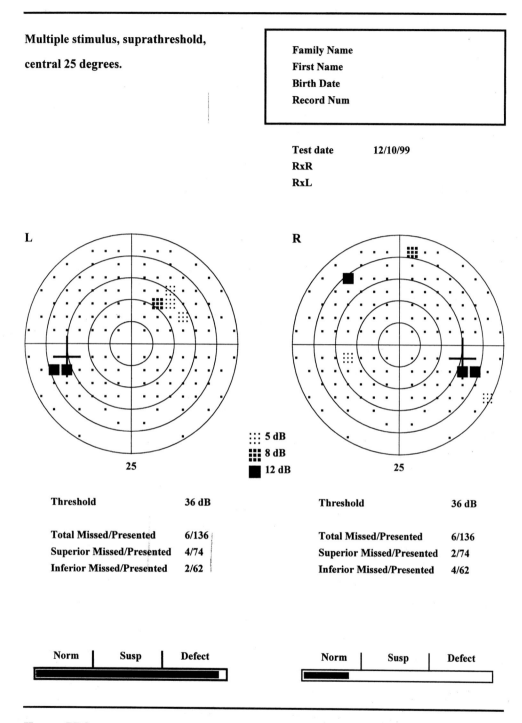

Fig. 9.9   *The right eye has four scattered non–blind spot misses while the left eye has four clustered non–blind spot misses. Note how the scale at the bottom of the printout, which represents the output of the scoring algorithm, indicates normal for the right eye and defect for the left eye. This scoring algorithm includes a cluster analysis routine.*

$$\text{Mean defect} = \frac{1}{n}\sum_{i=1}^{n}(z_i - x_i)$$

z_i = Age corrected normal value at test location i

n = Number of test locations

x_i = Measured sensitivity at test location i

Fig. 9.10 *Formula for the calculation of mean defect, Octopus.*

by any kind of visual field defect although it is more sensitive to generalized depression than to small local defects. On its own mean defect is neither very sensitive nor specific to glaucomatous loss (Enger and Sommer, 1987). Its greatest value is not in the detection of abnormality but in the long term monitoring of patients with established loss.

An important parameter in the calculation of the mean defect is the set of normal values to which the results are compared. Any error in this data set will produce apparent errors in all patients with normal visual fields. The relatively small data set used to calculate normal values has subsequently been shown to be in error by 0.2 dB. The results from a normal population will, therefore, be centred on a value of 0.2 dB rather than 0 dB. The standard deviation of mean defect values is 1.5 dB (Flammer *et al.*, 1985). We should therefore expect 68% of normal patients to have values between −1.30 dB and +1.70 dB and 95% to lie between −2.80 dB and +3.30 dB.

Loss variation and corrected loss variation. This index is designed to give a measure of local loss. Flammer *et al.* (1985) recognized that local loss would result in low sensitivity measures at certain locations in the field and that the computed defect (the difference between the measured sensitivity and the age-matched normal value) of these areas would be large. There would, therefore, be an increase in the total range of defect values. They chose to represent the range of defect values with a statistic called variance. The variance is calculated in three stages:

1. The mean defect is calculated (see above).
2. The mean defect is subtracted from the measured defect at each tested location.
3. These values are then squared (to remove negative values), added together and divided by the total number of test locations (see Figure 9.11).

Flammer *et al.*, (1985) recognized that this measure of dispersion, which they called loss variation, included a component which was due to normal variability and as a consequence it is unlikely ever to be zero. To overcome this problem they proposed that loss variation should be corrected by a value that represented the patient's normal variation. By subtracting the normal variance from the loss variation they produced a new index, called corrected loss variation, the value of which is centred around zero (see Figure 9.11).

The patient's normal variance is calculated by taking repeat measures of the threshold (usually at a few test locations) and looking at the differences between the repeat measures. Short-term fluctuation is the square root of the patient's estimated normal variation, (see below for more details). Hence corrected loss variation is calculated by subtracting the square of the short-term fluctuation from the loss variance.

The normal values for corrected loss variation are 1.50 with a standard deviation of 2.60 dB^2 (Flammer *et al.*, 1985).

Short-term fluctuation. It is well known that if you measure the eye's sensitivity at the same location twice it is unlikely that you will get the exact same result; there is a degree of variability in the results. It is also recognized that in glaucoma there is an increase in the amount of variability. Short-term fluctuation is a measure of the scatter that occurs during a single visual field examination. This index is obtained by repeating the threshold measures at some or all of the test locations, (in the majority of cases, programs 31 and 32, two

$$\text{Loss variance} = \frac{1}{n-1}\sum_{i=1}^{m}(x_i + \text{MD} - z_i)^2$$

$\dfrac{\text{Corrected loss}}{\text{variance}}$ = Loss variance − (Short term fluctuation)^2

z_i = Age corrected normal value at test location i

x_i = Measured sensitivity at test location i

MD = Mean defect

n = Number of test locations

Fig. 9.11 *Formula for the calculation of loss variance and corrected loss variance, Octopus.*

$$\frac{\text{Short-term}}{\text{fluctuation}} = \frac{\text{Total variance}}{\text{Number of double determinations}}$$

$$= \left[\frac{1}{m} \sum_{i=1}^{m} \frac{\sum_{k=1}^{R}(x_{ik} - \bar{x}_i)^2}{R-1} \right]^{\frac{1}{2}}$$

$\bar{x}_i = $ Mean sensitivity at location i

$x_{ik} = $ Sensitivity at location i repetition k

$m = $ Number of locations with repeat measures

$R = $ Number of repetitions, normally 2

Fig. 9.12 *Formula for the calculation of short-term fluctuation, Octopus.*

measures of the threshold are taken at 10 different locations). The results are then analysed in the following way:

1. The average threshold is calculated for each location in which repeat measures are available.
2. The average is subtracted from each of the measurements at each location, and the result squared to remove negative values.
3. These values are then added together to give the sum of the squares for each location where repeat measures have been taken. This value is then divided by the number of repeat values minus 1 (in the majority of cases where only two measures are taken the value is divided by 1).
4. The sum of the squares for each location are then added together and divided by the total number of locations at which repeat measures have been taken to give a measure of subject variance.
5. This measure of variance is then square rooted to give the index 'short-term fluctuation' (see Figure 9.12).

Bebie curve. The Bebie curve is not strictly speaking a quantification system in that it does not reduce the graphical results obtained from an examination into one number or a group of numbers. The curve is an alternative form of graphically representing the data from a full-threshold examination that has certain advantages for result interpretation. The ability to

produce a Bebie curve is built into the software of the Octopus perimeters (1-2-3 and 101).

A problem encountered with the use of the 3 indices described above is that measures of overall loss (mean defect and mean deviation) are also sensitive to local changes. If a patient has a scotoma that increases in depth or size then not only will the variance indices change (Corrected Loss Variance and Corrected Pattern Standard Deviation) but also the indices designed to measure overall changes. To overcome this problem Bebie *et al.*, (1989); (see also Kaufmann and Flammer, 1989) developed a technique of graphically representing the data which they called a Bebie curve. With a Bebie curve the individual defect values are ranked according to depth and then plotted, in rank order, along the x-axis, the y-axis being the defect level (see Figure 9.13). A patient with only diffuse loss will have a curve that shows a relatively constant deviation from the norm. A patient with local loss will have a curve that follows the normal range until it gets to the right-hand side where the large individual defects are plotted. It then shows large deviations from the norm. Changes in overall loss and localized loss will have different effects upon the Bebie curve. Changes in overall loss will result in a lowering of the curve, while increases in the size of a scotoma will produce a shift, to the left, of the sharp line demarcating between normal and defective test points.

Humphrey indices

Clearly, a very important parameter in the calculation of mean defect and corrected loss variance is the aged matched normal sensitivity values. In the Octopus instrument certain assumptions concerning these values have been made:

1. That the slopes of the sensitivity profiles do not change with age.
2. That with age the overall sensitivity decreases at a rate of 1 dB per decade.
3. That the variability in threshold measures is constant across the visual field.

In developing a similar set of indices for the Humphrey Visual Field Analyzer, Heijl *et al.*, (1987) collected data from a large population of normal patients and produced a set of normal values which did not make the above assumptions. This data set

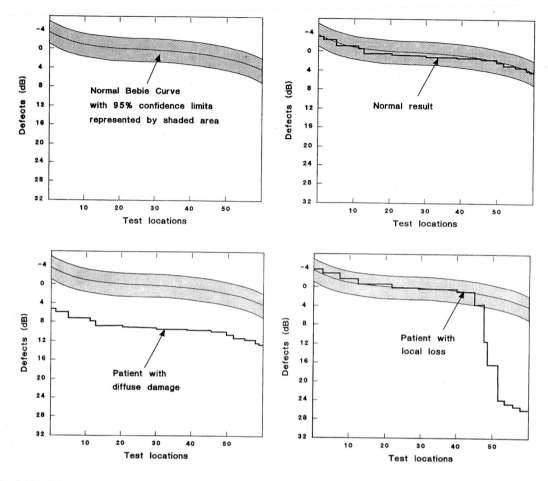

Fig. 9.13 *Bebie curves.*

has been incorporated into the Humphrey Statpac package for the purposes of calculating the indices, mean deviation, corrected pattern standard deviation and short-term fluctuation.

Mean deviation. From Figure 9.14 it can be seen that the Humphrey calculation of mean deviation differs from the Octopus calculation of mean defect by the addition of a measure of variance. The effect of this addition is to weight each measure of deviation according to the normal degree of variance found at that location. Measures that come from locations in which there is little variance are given greater importance in the calculation of the index than those that come from areas in which there is a great deal of variance. The similarities between the calculation of mean defect and mean deviation can be appreciated if one makes the

variance term in the mean deviation formula a constant. In this case the equation for mean deviation reduces to that of mean defect.

$$\text{Mean deviation} = \left[\frac{1}{n} \sum_{i=1}^{n} \frac{(z_i - x_i)}{s_{1i}^2} \right] \Big/ \left[\frac{1}{n} \sum_{i=1}^{n} \frac{1}{s_{1i}^2} \right]$$

$z_i = $ Age corrected normal value at test location i

$n = $ Number of test locations

$x_i = $ Measured sensitivity at test location i

$s_{1i}^2 = $ Variance of normal field measurements

     at location i

Fig. 9.14 *Formula for the calculation of mean deviation, Humphrey.*

$$\left[\begin{array}{c}\text{Pattern}\\\text{standard}\\\text{deviation}\end{array}\right]^2 = \left[\frac{1}{n-1}\sum_{i=1}^{m}\frac{(x_i + \text{MD} - z_i)^2}{s_{1i}^2}\right] \times \left[\frac{1}{n}\sum_{i=1}^{m}s_{1i}^2\right]$$

$$\left[\begin{array}{c}\text{Corrected}\\\text{pattern}\\\text{standard}\\\text{deviation}\end{array}\right]^2 = \left[\begin{array}{c}\text{Pattern}\\\text{standard}\\\text{deviation}\end{array}\right]^2 - k \times (\text{Short-term fluctuation})^2$$

z_i = Age corrected normal value at test location i

x_i = Measured sensitivity at test location i

MD = Mean deviation

n = Number of test locations

s_{1i}^2 = Variance of normal field measurements at location i

k = Constant (<1) to adjust for non-uniform fluctuation

Fig. 9.15 *Formula for the calculation of pattern standard deviation and corrected pattern standard deviation, Humphrey.*

Pattern standard deviation and corrected pattern standard deviation. Pattern standard deviation and corrected pattern standard deviation are indices designed to reflect the amount of local field loss in eyes with, or suspected of having, glaucoma. In many ways these indices are similar to those of loss variance and corrected loss variance as developed by Flammer *et al.*, (1985) for the Octopus. There are two major differences:

1. In the Humphrey instrument, Heijl *et al.*, (1987) have chosen to use standard deviation rather than variance to represent local loss. The standard deviation is, in fact, the square root of the variance. It is often preferred to variance because it gives a measure of dispersion in the same units as the variable.
2. Each location used to calculate the pattern standard deviation has been weighted according to the normal degree of variance found at that location. Measures from locations in which the variance is low have a more significant input to the index than those from locations in which the variance is normally high.

Pattern standard deviation can be thought of as the square root of loss variance that has been weighted

$$\text{Short-term fluctuation} = \left[\left[\frac{1}{m}\sum_{i=1}^{m}s_{2i}^2\right] \times \left[\frac{1}{m}\sum_{i=1}^{m}\frac{\sum_{k=1}^{R}(x_{ik}-\bar{x}_i)^2}{R-1}\right]\right]^{1/2}$$

s_{2i}^2 = Normal intra-test variance at point i

$\bar{x}$ = Mean sensitivity at location i

x_{ik} = Sensitivity at location i, repetition k

m = Number of locations with repeat measures

R = Number of repetitions, normally 2

Fig. 9.16 *Formula for the calculation of short-term fluctuation, Humphrey.*

according to the normally occurring scatter that occurs at each retinal location.

Pattern standard deviation, as well as loss variation, contains a component that results from the normally occurring scatter in any threshold measure. The normal scatter can be estimated by repeat measurements. Corrected pattern standard deviation is the pattern standard deviation minus the estimated scatter as represented by the index short-term fluctuation (see below). It is computed by subtracting the square of the short-term fluctuation multiplied by a constant k (>1) from the square of the pattern standard deviation and then taking the square root of the result (see Figure 9.15). The constant k is 'to adjust for the non-uniform fluctuation pattern' (Heijl *et al.*, 1987).

Short-term fluctuation. The short-term fluctuation index on the Humphrey instrument is very similar to that found in the Octopus. It differs in that the individual sum of the squares measures for each location are weighted according to the normally occurring variance at that location (see Figure 9.16).

Glaucoma hemifield test (GHT). The GHT (Sommer *et al.*, 1987; Åsman and Heijl 1992a) is designed to detect rather than quantify visual field defects. It is based upon a common characteristic of glaucomatous defects, i.e. vertical asymmetry between the superior and inferior hemifields. The GHT looks at the asymmetry in pattern deviation probability values between five areas in the superior field and their mirror images in the inferior field (see Figure

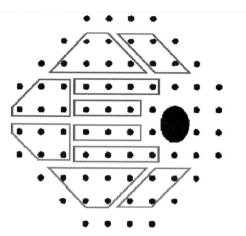

Fig. 9.17 *Regions of the central field used in the glaucoma hemifield test.*

beyond the 99% limit for normals in any of the five sector pairs.

3. Borderline. The asymmetry is beyond the 97% limit for normal in any sector pair.
4. General reduction in sensitivity. The general height is below the 0.5% limit for normals.
5. Within normal limits.

The GHT has been evaluated by both Åsman and Heijl (1992b) and by Katz *et al.*, (1996).

Its improved performance, in comparison to global indices, is attributed to its use of some of the spatial information contained within the visual field chart. (See p. 130 for details of other techniques, which retain the spatial information.)

9.17). It uses a database to compare the asymmetries with those from a normal population and then establishes whether or not they are outside of the normal limits.

The GHT produces a series of different categorical outputs:

1. Abnormally high sensitivity. The general height of the field is beyond the 99.5% limit for normals. General height is calculated from the deviation values being the seventh highest value from the 24-2 set of data points.
2. Outside normal limits. The asymmetry is

Box plots. In addition to plotting the three indices described above, the Humphrey Visual Field Analyzer also represents its results in a box plot (see Figures 9.18, 9.19 and 9.20). Each box plot, there being one for each visit, displays the distribution of threshold values across the whole field. The most sensitive point is represented by the top of the 'T' while the least sensitive point is represented by the bottom of the inverted 'T'. The top of the box is the 85th percentile, i.e. 85% of the tested locations had a sensitivity below this level, while the bottom of the box represents the 15th percentile, i.e. 15% of the tested locations had a sensitivity below this value. The three bars near the middle of the box represent the 50th percentile.

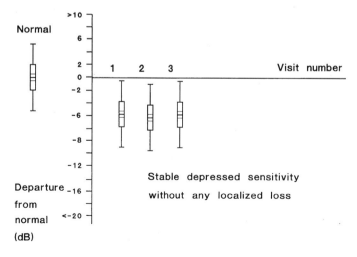

Fig. 9.18 *Box plots from a patient with stable depressed sensitivity.*

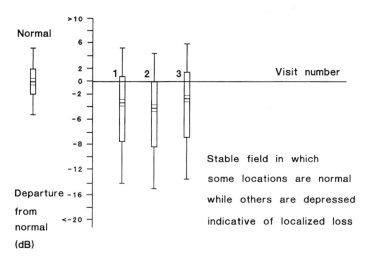

Fig. 9.19 *Box plots from a patient with stable localized loss.*

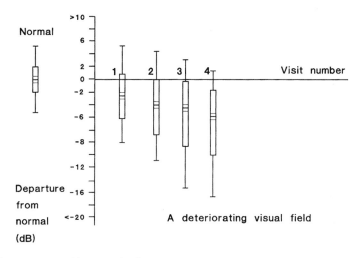

Fig. 9.20 *Box plots from a patient with progressive loss.*

A normal patient should give a result similar to that shown on the left-hand side of each diagram; the three bars should be centred around 0, the most sensitive point approximately 5 dB above 0 and the least sensitive point approximately 5 dB below. If the patient has a diffuse loss then the box plot will be shifted down (see Figure 9.18), while a localized loss will be represented by an elongation of the box towards the defect region (see Figure 9.19).

One of the great assets of box plots is their ability to display the results from several examinations at the same time and allow the perimetrist to establish whether there is any trend (see Figure 9.20).

Practical differences between Octopus and Humphrey indices

The Humphrey modifications to the three indices (mean defect, loss variance and fluctuation) initially proposed by Flammer *et al.*, (1985) reduce the normal range of values and thereby increase the capability of the indices to separate normal from abnormal. In practice the additional sophistication of the computations does not have a major effect upon their utility (Funkhouser and Fankhauser, 1990).

The normal range of values is still large and the indices do not take into account factors such as the clustering of missed stimuli. Their greatest strength is more to do with the monitoring of established loss rather than in the initial detection of defects, although recent reports indicate that the inherent variability in these techniques makes it very difficult to detect trends (Chauhan *et al.*, 1990).

Empirical cut-off and grading systems

An alternative way of differentiating between eyes which have glaucomatous visual field loss and those which do not is to apply a simple set of criteria such as three or more contiguous test locations with at least 5 dB reduction of threshold sensitivity compared to age-corrected normal values. There are, obviously, a large number of criteria that could be used. Some groups have excluded locations that are at the edge of the visual field while others base their definition of a defective visual field on defects that are replicated in a second examination.

These systems can be extended to provide a visual field score that can be monitored over time. One of the most widely used scoring systems was that devised for the Advanced Glaucoma Intervention Study (AGIS) (AGIS Study Investigators, 1994). This scoring system is based upon the number and depth of depressions from age match normal results from the full-threshold 24-2 test program. The scoring system also takes into account a number of reliability parameters such as the number of fixation losses, false positives, false negatives and the number of questions asked (this goes up when the visual field result is more complex). The score ranges from 0 (no defect) to 20 (end stage). A similar scoring system has been developed for the Collaborative Initial Glaucoma Treatment Study (CIGTS) (see Katz, 1999).

These scoring systems are based upon clinical experience rather than an analysis of visual field data.

Quantification of asymmetry

All of the quantification systems described so far, be they for kinetic, suprathreshold static or full-threshold static techniques, treat each eye independently and do not take into account the similarity that normally exists between the two eyes. A normal patient who has a slightly depressed sensitivity in one eye invariably has a slightly depressed sensitivity in the other.

While many pathological conditions are binocular, they invariably affect one eye before the other. For example, in an analysis conducted by Henson *et al.*, (1986) it was found that over 90% of patients with glaucoma had significant asymmetries between the two eyes.

In theory, improved detection rates can, therefore, be obtained by analysing the differences between the scores of the right and left eyes. To do this the results from both the right and left eyes of a population of normal patients must first be calculated. The right eye's score is then subtracted from the left eye's score, all the values made positive and a distribution of the differences formed. The differences between the right and left eyes of any new patient can then be compared to this distribution to see if it falls within the normal range (Henson *et al.*, 1986; Sponsel *et al.*, 1987).

Artificial neural networks

Another, totally different, form of visual field analysis, which has recently received attention, involves the use of computer programs known collectively as artificial neural networks. Artificial neural network programs have the ability to learn and subsequently recognize patterns, i.e. they are pattern recognition programs.

Several researchers have already applied neural network programs to visual field data to test whether or not the networks can recognize and differentiate characteristic patterns of visual field loss. In practice a neural network is initially taught, through repetition, to recognize various types of visual field loss. These defects are incorporated into what is called a training set of data. After the network has reached a high degree of classification accuracy with the training set of data it is presented with new field data and asked to classify it according to what it has 'learnt'. From what has just been said, you can probably gather why the term neural network is used. These programs are designed to mimic the learning process found within the neural networks of the brain; they are often described as 'biologically inspired programs'.

Various research papers have reported that neural networks can achieve over 90% classification accuracy (see Spenceley *et al.*, 1994), which is probably very close to the degree of accuracy that trained clinicians would reach given the same type of task.

One of the attractions of neural networks is that there is no need to define the different classifications, that is left to the neural network to work out.

You may be wondering whether the role of interpreting visual field defects is soon to be taken over by the computer. Do not worry, neural networks currently have some severe limitations. Most importantly, they do not learn from experience. If they are not given every possible type of defect in their training set they might never learn to correctly classify certain types of defect. Contrast this with the case of a student who, after making a few mistakes, would modify his or her future decisions and hopefully improve their performance. This limitation in neural networks means that the training set has to be very carefully selected to accurately represent each of the classification groups. This is a surprisingly difficult task. However, it must be said in support of neural networks that they are very much in their infancy and today's limitations may well be overcome in the not too distant future.

Indices for monitoring the progression of field loss

All of the techniques described so far, be they for kinetic, suprathreshold static or full-threshold static strategies, quantify the extent of loss in a single visual field examination. Now, clearly, these numbers/indices can be monitored over a period of time to establish whether the visual field defect is progressing, stable or improving.

A problem that arises when utilizing indices in this way is that of establishing whether the change in the values is significant. Remember each visual field score is subject to a certain amount of variability. If you measure the same eye over and over again you do not necessarily get the same result. How do you know, when you have two visual field records, taken during separate visits of the same patient, whether the differences in the visual field scores are the result of this normal variability or represent a real change in the field defect?

In an attempt to overcome this problem there have, over the past few years, been a series of proposals in which statistical tests are used to evaluate progression. The major ones are:

- Paired t-test.
- Linear regression.
- Change probability

Paired t-test

The Octopus system uses a software package (Delta program) which employs a paired t-test to compare mean sensitivities (Werner *et al.*, 1988). This program can be used to look at all test locations or only those that are deemed to be abnormal. It compares the mean sensitivity of the first record with that from the last for each location and computes the mean difference per test location. (Note that this technique is only appropriate for comparing two sets of data. When more than two sets are available the intermediate sets are either ignored or averaged with the other sets.) If the mean difference is significantly different ($P > 0.05$), the visual field is considered to have changed. An evaluation of this method of detecting visual field changes was carried out by Hills and Johnson (1988). They used real visual field records into which they inserted a scotoma of known depth and size and then computed how this would affect the t-test values. They found that while the test was very sensitive to small changes in the entire visual field it was relatively insensitive to small to moderate scotoma (<18 degrees in diameter), even when the sensitivity loss within the scotoma was as great as 35 dB. They concluded that it had limited clinical utility.

Linear regression

Linear regression is a statistical technique which establishes the best fitting straight line to a series of visual field tests taken over a period of time. If the best fitting line has a negative gradient, i.e. it is going downhill, then the visual field is deteriorating. If it is flat (gradient 0) then the field is stable and if the gradient is positive it is improving. One of the advantages of the linear regression technique is that it not only gives you the gradient but also its confidence limits. By adding and subtracting the confidence limits to the gradient we can establish whether or not the gradient is significantly different from zero (if the value plus and minus the confidence limits includes zero then it is not significantly different). The magnitude of the confidence limits will vary with the amount of data and the variability in the data. Linear regression techniques also have the advantage of being

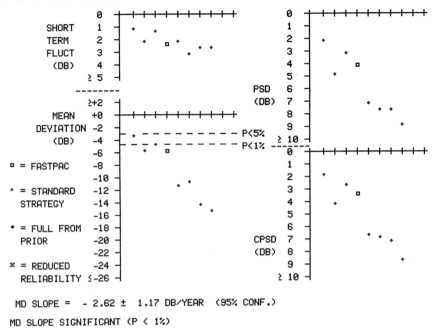

Fig. 9.21 *Results from a regression analysis of the global index mean deviation (MD). Also shown are the indices short-term fluctuation (Short-Term Fluct), pattern standard deviation (PSD) and corrected pattern standard deviation (CPSD). Data has been collected from eight visual field records taken with the Humphrey Visual Field Analyzer. In this example the regression analysis shows a significant deterioration.*

able to utilize more than two sets of data (to perform a linear regression you need a minimum of three sets of data). They are thus more appropriate for looking at long-term trends in data.

Linear regression can be applied to:

- global measures of the visual field,
- regional measures of the visual field or
- individual test locations (pointwise analysis).

Figure 9.21 shows the application of linear regression to the global measures obtained from a Humphrey Visual Field Analyzer. The patient has undergone eight visual field examinations over a period of 5 years. The plots show that the index Mean Deviation is getting worse as are the indices Pattern Standard Deviation (PSD) and Corrected Pattern Standard Deviation (CPSD). At the bottom there are two statements which come from a regression analysis applied to the Mean Deviation data. One tells us that the slope of the best fitting straight line has a gradient of $-2.62 \, dB/year$, i.e. the field is deteriorating. It also gives the 95% confidence limits for the slope (± 1.17) This means that we can be 95% sure that

the gradient lies between -1.45 and $-3.79 \, dB/year$. As these values do not include zero then we can state that there is a significant deterioration (at the 5% level). One further statistic is provided. It states that the slope is significant at $P < 1\%$. This means that there is a less than 1% chance that slope is not negative. This example comes from a straightforward case in which there is plenty of good data from which we can draw our conclusions.

Figure 9.22 gives the results from another patient in which the decision is not so straightforward. In this case there are only six visual field records and the results are much more variable. Because of this variability the regression analysis concludes that the slope is not significantly different from zero at the 5% level. The gradient of the regression line is negative (-0.38) but the 95% confidence limits (± 0.84) when added to the gradient would include a value of zero.

Werner *et al.*, (1988) and O'Brien and Schwartz (1990) recognized that the use of global indices, which analyse the results from all test locations, may conceal significant changes in one part of the visual field. They suggested that it might be better if

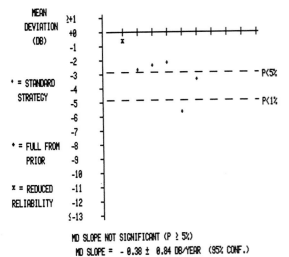

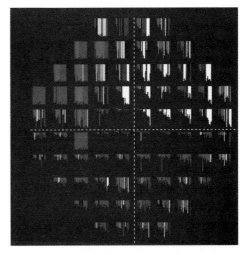

Fig. 9.22 *Result from a regression analysis of the global index mean deviation on six visual field records taken with a Humphrey Visual Field Analyzer. Note that the data show a declining MD value but that this is not significant because the confidence limits when added to the MD slope include 0. The large confidence limits are due to the large amount of variability in this set of data.*

Fig. 9.23 *The result from a pointwise regression analysis using the software package 'Progressor'. The vertical bars at each test location give the sensitivity at each visit: the longer the bar the more defective the test location. The colour of the bars gives the significance: the hotter the colour the more significant the change.*

different areas of the visual field were analysed separately. They chose areas which included between five and nine test locations, on the basis of the distribution of the ganglion cell nerve fibres. Their results demonstrated that in certain cases significant progressive loss could be detected in patients whose overall analysis showed no significant progressive loss, i.e. that regional analysis is, on occasions, more sensitive than global analysis.

The process was taken one step further by a group of researchers at the Institute of Ophthalmology, London (see Fitzke *et al.*, 1996). They have developed the technique of pointwise linear regression, where each test location is subjected to regression analysis. Given that there are often 52 test locations, this type of analysis would yield 52 regression equations and 52 sets of confidence limits. Clearly, one of the major problems with this type of analysis is displaying all the data in a way that facilitates the recognition of progressive loss. The group at the Institute of Ophthalmology found a graphical solution to this problem (see Figure 9.23). At each test location a vertical bar represents the results of each visual field test. The length of the bar corresponds to the sensitivity: the longer the bar, the

lower the sensitivity. The colour of the bar relates to the significance of the regression slope (rate of change). Undamaged locations are seen as a series of short grey bars, damaged, but stable, locations are seen as a series of long grey bars and locations with progressive loss are seen as a series of lengthening bars whose colour becomes hotter as the change becomes more and more significant. This form of analysis is available in the stand-alone Progressor software package. One of the advantages of displaying the data in this way is that it retains the spatial information contained within the visual field chart. The clinician can ascertain whether or not any progressive changes are close to fixation or at the edge of the visual field where they may have been influenced by artefacts such as a droopy upper lid.

When a patient with glaucoma is being reviewed in the clinic the clinician needs to decide whether or not the visual field is getting worse and whether or not there should be a change in the treatment. The clinician must make a decision on the overall status of the visual field. When using pointwise analysis it is necessary to have a set of criteria for deciding when there is some overall change, e.g. slope worse than $-1\,dB$ per year for inner locations and greater than $-2\,dB$ per year for edge locations ($P < 0.05$) at one or more test locations.

Regression analysis, while having the advantage of being able to use the data from a long series of measurements, has a number of shortcomings. The most important of these is that the analysis is very dependent upon there being a fairly large amount of data. You cannot do a regression analysis when you only have two visual field results and your ability to accurately predict the gradient improves the more data you have. Several research groups have concluded that you really need about six visual field results before you can reliably calculate the gradient of the regression line.

Change probability

In a clinical environment the question most often asked of the perimetrist is 'has there been any change?'. To reply that we cannot tell, even after the patient has been tested for over 30 minutes, until we have collected some more data is not really very helpful. What is needed is a quantification technique that can compare the current visual field result with a previous one and to tell the perimetrist which, if any, test locations have changed. Change probability analysis is a technique that does just that. It uses a set of baseline data which is very often the average of two previous visual field records and then compares the current result with the baseline at each test location and computes whether or not it has changed by a significant amount.

This type of analysis is similar, in many ways, to the total and pattern deviation probability maps that were described in Chapter 3, p. 37. It differs in that rather than establish whether or not the data at each location is significantly different from normal it establishes whether or not it is significantly different from the baseline value which, of course, could already be abnormal.

It is well established that the variability in threshold estimates is dependent upon the threshold. The lower the threshold the more variable the results. Change probability analysis needs to take this into account. In the Humphrey Visual Field Analyzer a database from patients with stable glaucomatous visual field loss is used to empirically establish whether or not any change is significant. The results from this analysis are displayed as a map in which different symbols represent the significance level of any change. Again, when interpreting the data from a

probability change analysis perimetrists normally apply a set of criteria such as two or more locations showing change at $P < 0.05$ on two separate occasions.

Change probability analysis is very sensitive to information stored within its database of stable glaucomatous eyes. Small differences in the database can have significant effects upon the distribution, especially at its extremes. It is the extremes of the distribution that are used in the calculation of change probability.

Conclusions on quantifying progression

In general, the use of statistics to evaluate the progression of visual field defects is fraught with both statistical and clinical problems, although in their defence the results are often more consistent than are the clinical impressions obtained from a number of ophthalmologists (Werner *et al.*, 1988).

One of the most difficult problems associated with progression is that of getting a technique that is both sensitive enough to detect change at an early stage and yet which also retains a high level of specificity. In many research projects the solution to this problem has been to have a sensitive set of criteria which, when met, trigger further data collection. Progression is then defined upon the results from both visual field tests rather than a single one, e.g. two or more of the same test locations showing change on two occasions. These definitions are rarely based upon any formal analysis of visual field data but do have a good deal of empirical support.

CONCLUSIONS

Now that we have reached the end of this chapter what conclusions can be drawn about the efficiency and value of quantifying visual field data?

There is no doubt that for measuring the extent of field loss, for purposes such as litigation, the current systems are perfectly adequate.

It is also true to say that as far as detecting abnormality is concerned, quantification systems have reached a level of sophistication which make them of considerable value to the clinician. Yet it should always be remembered that these systems are only a guide and not a definitive statement. Every clinician can cite examples of a quantification system that suggests the existence of a defect when the patient is known to have a perfectly normal visual field, e.g. refraction scotomas.

The value of quantification systems in being able to monitor the progression of an individual's visual field loss is still, however, severely limited. Reliable estimates of any trend usually require several sets of data taken over extensive periods of time. Part of the problem lies in the very nature of the visual field results, which are subject to a large degree of variability.

The above statements are not meant to imply that the current quantification systems have no role to play in the monitoring of visual field defects. In trials that include significant numbers of patients, overall trends can be detected and the results from different treatment regimes compared. The point to be made here is that in individual patients the results from these systems should be treated with care.

We should not, however, give up on quantification systems. Decision making in glaucoma needs to be made on the basis of long-term predictions that realistically can only be made by modelling visual field trends.

REFERENCES

AGIS Study Investigators (1994) Advanced glaucoma intervention study. 2. Visual field test scoring and reliability. *Ophthalmology*, **101**, 1445–1455.

Åsman P. and Heijl A. (1992a) Glaucoma hemifield test. Automated visual field evaluation. *Arch Ophthalmol*, **110**, 812–819.

Åsman P. and Heijl A. (1992b) Evaluation of methods for automated hemifield analysis in perimetry. *Arch Ophthalmol*, **110**, 820–826.

Bebie H., Flammer J. and Bebie Th. (1989) Cumulative defect curve, separation of local and diffuse components of visual field damage. *Graef Arch Clin Exp Ophthalmol*, **227**, 9–12.

Birch M.K., Wishart P.K. and O Donnell N.P. (1995) Determining progressive visual field loss in serial Humphrey visual fields. *Ophthalmology*, **102**, 1227–1235.

Capris P., Gandolfo E., Camoriano G.P. and Zingirian M. (1987) Kinetic visual field indices. In *Perimetry Update 1988/89* (ed. Heijl A.). Kugler & Ghedini, Amsterdam, pp. 223–227.

Chauhan B.C., Drance S.M. and Douglas G.R. (1990) The use of visual field indices in detecting changes in the visual field in glaucoma. *Invest Ophthalmol Vis Sci*, **31**, 512–520.

Enger C. and Sommer A. (1987) Recognizing glaucomatous field loss with the Humphrey Statpac. *Arch Ophthalmol*, **105**, 1355–1357.

Esterman B. (1967) Grid for scoring visual fields. I Tangent screen. *Arch Ophthalmol*, **77**, 780–786.

Esterman B. (1968) Grid for scoring visual fields. II Perimeter. *Arch Ophthalmol*, **79**, 400–406.

Esterman B. (1982) Functional scoring of the binocular field. *Ophthalmol*, **89**, 1226–1234.

Esterman B., Blanche E., Wallach M. and Bonelli A. (1985) Computerised scoring of the functional field. *Doc Ophthalmol Proc Ser*, **42**, 333–339.

Fitzke F.W., Hitchins R.A., Poinoosawmy D., McNaught A.I. and Crabb D.P. (1996) Analysis of visual field progression in glaucoma. *Br J Ophthalmol*, **80**, 40–48.

Flammer J., Drance S.M., Augustiny L. and Funkhouser A. (1985) Quantification of glaucomatous visual field defects with automated perimetry. *Invest Ophthalmol Vis Sci*, **26**, 176–181.

Funkhouser A.T. and Fankhauser F. (1990) A comparison of the mean defect and mean deviation indices within the central 28 degrees of the glaucomatous visual field. *Jpn J Ophthalmol*, **34**, 414–420.

Hart W.M. and Hartz R.K. (1981) Computer processing of visual field data. *Arch Ophthalmol*, **99**, 128–132.

Heijl A., Lindgren G. and Olsson J. (1987) A package for the statistical analysis of visual fields. *Doc Ophthalmol Proc Series* **49**, 153–168.

Henson D.B. and Bryson H. (1987) Clinical results with the Henson–Hamblin CFS2000. *Doc Ophthalmol Proc Series*, **49**, 233–238.

Henson D.B. and Dix S.M. (1984) Evaluation of the Friedmann Visual Field Analyser Mark II. Part 1. Results from a normal population. *Br J Ophthalmol*, **68**, 458–462.

Henson D.B., Dix S.M. and Oborne A.C. (1984) Evaluation of the Friedmann Visual Field Analyser Mark II. Part 2. Results from a population with induced visual field defects. *Br J Ophthalmol*, **68**, 463–467.

Henson D.B., Hobley A., Chauhan B., Sponsel W. and Dallas N. (1986) Importance of visual field score and asymmetry in the detection of glaucoma. *Am J Optom Physiol Optics*, **63**, 714–723.

Hills J.F. and Johnson C.A. (1988) Evaluation of the t-test as a method of detecting visual field change. *Ophthalmology*, **95**, 261–266.

Hirsch J. (1985) Statistical analysis in computerised perimetry. In *Computerised Visual Fields: What They Are and How to Use Them* (eds Whalen W.R. and Spaeth G.L.). Slack Inc, Thorofare, NJ.

Hobley A. (1986) *The quantification of visual fields and the detection of chronic open angle glaucoma.* MSc thesis, University of Wales.

Holmin C. and Krakau C.E.T. (1982) Regression analysis of the central visual field in chronic glaucoma cases. *Acta Ophthalmol*, **60**, 267–274.

Katz J. (1999) Scoring systems for measuring progression of visual field loss in clinical trials of glaucoma treatment. *Ophthalmology*, **106**, 391–395.

Katz J., Quigley H.A. and Sommer A. (1996) Detection of incident field loss using the glaucoma hemifield test. *Ophthalmology*, **103**, 657–663.

Kaufmann H. and Flammer J. (1989) Clinical experiences with the Bebie curve. In *Perimetry Update 1988/89* (ed. Heijl A.). Kugler & Ghedini, Amsterdam, pp. 235–238.

Mikelberg F.S., Schultzer M., Drance S.M. and Lau W. (1986) The rate of progression of scotoma in glaucoma. *Am J Ophthalmol*, **101**, 1–6.

O Brien C. and Schwartz B. (1990) The visual field in chronic open angle glaucoma: the rate of change in different regions of the field. *Eye*, **4**, 557–562.

Pe'er J., Zajicek G. and Barzel I. (1983) Computerised evaluation of visual fields. *Br J Ophthalmol*, **67**, 50–53.

Schultz J.S., Werner E.B., Krupin T. *et al.* (1987) Intraocular pressure and visual field defects following argon laser trabeculoplasty in chronic open-angle glaucoma. *Ophthalmol*, **94**, 553–557.

Schultzer M., Mikelberg F.S. and Drance S.M. (1987) A study of the central and peripheral isopters in assessing visual field progression in the presence of paracentral scotoma measurements. *Br J Ophthalmol*, **71**, 422–427.

Shapiro L.R., Johnson C.A. and Kennedy R.L. (1989) A computer simulation procedure for static, kinetic, supra-threshold and heuristic perimetry. In *Perimetry Update 1988/89* (ed. Heijl A.). Kugler & Ghedini, Amsterdam, pp. 431–438.

Smith R. (1968) A comparison between medical and surgical treatment of glaucoma simplex. Results from a prospective study. *Trans Ophthalmol Soc Aust*, **27**, 17–29.

Sommer A., Enger C. and Witt K. (1987) Screening for glaucomatous visual field loss with automated threshold perimetry. *Am J Ophthalmol*, **103**, 681–684.

Spenceley S.E., Henson D.B. and Bull D.R. (1994) Visual field analysis using artificial neural networks. *Ophthalmic Physiol Opt*, **14**, 239–248.

Sponsel W.E., Hobley A., Henson D.B., Chauhan B.C. and Dallas N.L. (1987) Quantitative supra-threshold static perimetry; the value of field score and asymmetry analysis in the detection of chronic open angle glaucoma. *Doc Ophthalmol Proc Series*, **49**, 217–229.

Sponsel W.E., Hobley A.J., Williams A.H. and Dallas N.L. (1984) Glaucoma assessment by microcomputer. *Trans Ophthalmol Soc UK*, **104**, 100–105.

Werner E.B., Bishop K.I., Koelle J., Douglas G.R., LeBlanc R.P., Mills R.P., Schwartz B., Whalen W.R. and Wilensky J.T. (1988) A comparison of experienced clinical observers and statistical tests in detection of progressive visual field loss in glaucoma using automated perimetry. *Arch Ophthalmol*, **106**, 619–623.

10 Practical advice on how to conduct a visual field examination

INTRODUCTION

Now that all the theory has been dealt with and the decisions have been made about which strategy is to be used, it is time to give some practical advice on how to conduct a visual field examination.

One could easily be forgiven for thinking that when you buy a new instrument it will come with a manual telling you how to conduct an examination. After all, the manufacturers have designed the instrument with a particular type of examination in mind so why not tell you what it is!

Well, by and large this is indeed the case. Most instruments include an operator manual which, in addition to telling you how to unpack it, turn it on etc. also tells you how to conduct an examination. The problem lies in the fact that not all instrument suppliers provide such information and that in some instances the manuals are not well written or assume a good deal of prior knowledge.

This chapter starts with a general description of what you should do before you commence a visual field examination. The chapter will then go on to give some practical guidance on how to conduct a visual field examination under a series of headings which correspond to the most widely used examination strategies. At the beginning of each section there is a list of instruments that use this strategy. For more details on each of these instruments the reader is referred to Chapter 11.

In this chapter it will be assumed that you have an instrument manual and that you will not need details on how to present the stimuli, select a program etc.

One last word, it is important to realize that there are many different ways of examining the visual field and each clinic tends to have its own particular way of doing things. The techniques described here should, therefore, only be considered as recommended techniques rather than the only way of doing things.

PROCEDURE TO BE ADOPTED PRIOR TO ANY VISUAL FIELD EXAMINATION

The following checklist is designed to be used prior to every field examination to avoid those silly mistakes that seem to occur with sickening regularity, such as forgetting to use a correcting lens or forgetting to patch the eye not being tested.

1. Turn room lights out and background illuminator/instrument on. Do this at the beginning because it will give the maximum amount of time for the patient to adapt to the instrument's background intensity level. Give an extended time for adaptation if the patient has just undergone an ophthalmoscopic examination or if the instrument's background illumination is low.
2. Patch the eye not being examined.
3. Correct any refractive error, preferably with a perimetric lens set (see Chapter 5 for table of recommended corrections). Remember to use a near correction for patients over the age of 40. Correcting lenses are only needed when testing the central 30 degrees of the visual field. For peripheral testing all lenses and lens holders should be removed.
4. If you are using a correcting lens which is placed in a lens holder attached to the instrument then make sure that the patient's eye is as close as possible to the correcting lens, ensuring that the eye is centred to the lens.
5. Make sure that the patient is comfortable. At this stage it is often helpful if you tell the patient that they will be required to keep still for some time.
6. Instruct the patient as to the nature of the test and his/her particular task. This, of course, varies with the instrument being used but will normally include a demonstration of the test and should always include numerous reminders of the importance of maintaining fixation.

KINETIC STRATEGY FOR WALL MOUNTED TANGENT SCREENS (CENTRAL 30 DEGREES)

Bjerrum screen, Bausch & Lomb Autoplot, Fincham Sutcliffe Screener (with Juler scotometer)

With these instruments the patient is positioned at either 1 m or, occasionally, 2 m from the screen. None of the instruments listed above incorporates either a background illuminator or any facilities for setting the background luminance. It is simply left up to the perimetrist to sort this out individually. Details on the appropriate levels are often difficult to establish but the essential thing in any practice is to ensure that the background luminance is fixed at some known value that can be monitored over time. If you use this type of instrument it is essential that you invest in a light meter and in some form of background illuminator whose output can be controlled and set to a specific light meter reading.

1. Select target (usually a 2 mm white spot).
2. Demonstrate the blind spot making sure that the patient understands the nature of the test. To do this place the target in the blind spot and then move it towards the fixation point until it is seen. The approximate position of the blind spot is often marked on the screen; if not, it is normally at an eccentricity of 15 degrees and 1.5 degrees below the horizontal midline in the temporal field. Repeat this several times, demonstrating to the patient how the target may disappear and how important it is to keep the eye still and looking at the fixation point.
3. Plot the extent of the visual field. Take the target right out to the periphery where it cannot be seen and then gradually bring it in along each meridian (usually every 15 degrees) until it is seen. Mark this point on the field chart. Some practitioners recommend that the target be oscillated from side to side as it is brought in towards the fixation point. The exact rationale behind this is unclear but as I mentioned at the beginning of this chapter each clinic tends to have its own particular way of doing things and this is simply one example.
4. Look for scotoma. This can be conducted either as a separate phase of the examination or in

combination with (3). Starting from the point where the stimulus was first seen, continue to move it in towards the centre of the field, the patient having been instructed to report if the stimulus fades or disappears. In order to check the patient's responses the perimetrist should occasionally extinguish the target. On instruments that project their stimuli, such as the Bausch & Lomb Autoplot, this can be achieved by simply pressing a button. With the Bjerrum screen, which uses painted targets on the end of a black wand, it can be achieved by twirling the wand to expose its reverse side, which is usually dark. If the patient either fails to respond or is slow to report that the stimulus has disappeared then, with the target still extinguished, ask him whether or not he can see it. Then demonstrate to the patient that on occasions you will make it disappear and that he is to report, as soon as possible, when this happens. The frequency with which you perform this additional test should be based upon the patient's responses. Those patients who are slow or fail to recognize that the target has disappeared should be tested more frequently than those who respond quickly.

5. Mark on the chart any positions where the patient cannot see the stimulus.

6. Plot the extent of the blind spot and any scotoma by moving from non-seeing to seeing, i.e. moving from within the blind spot/scotoma to a point where it is first seen.

7. The examination can be repeated with different sized or coloured targets, although detailed quantification of defects is normally left to more sophisticated instruments where the parameters of the examination are under better control.

KINETIC STRATEGY FOR BOWL PERIMETERS
Goldmann perimeter, Tubingen perimeter, Zeiss perimeter

These three bowl perimeters are mechanically very sophisticated and can be used in a variety of different ways. Two commonly used strategies are:

(a) isopter plotting, including detecting and measuring the area of scotoma;

(b) profile perimetry.

Plotting isopters

1. Select target – I-2e (or its equivalent) is the most widely used one for patients with normal sensitivity. Brighter, or larger, stimuli might be necessary for patients with media opacities.

2. Present the stimulus in the central region of the field. This is to establish that (a) the stimulus can be seen at the centre of the field, i.e. that the patient's sensitivity is not severely depressed and (b) to train the subject.

3. Take the stimulus out to the peripheral field, >60 degrees eccentricity, and then move it radially towards the centre at a speed of approximately 3–5 degrees per second. As soon as the patient reports the target seen, stop moving it and mark the chart at the position where it was first seen. It is important to monitor the patient's fixation while moving the stimulus. This is usually achieved by direct viewing of the patient's eye through an integral telescope.

4. Move the stimulus back out 10–15 degrees and then move it to an adjacent meridian (15 degrees away). Repeat above along all 24 meridians.

5. Now repeat the whole process with a different stimulus, usually the I-4e or its equivalent.

6. Complete the record chart by connecting up all the points for a given stimulus with a line indicating which stimulus was used (see Figure 10.1).

7. To detect scotoma, within the bounds of an isopter, statically present the stimuli used to plot the isopters at a series of different locations. The stimulus should be presented for approximately 1 second and the patient's responses noted. If the patient fails to see the stimulus then the area of defect should be investigated further (see below). The number of static spot checks will vary with the level of suspicion that the perimetrist already has.

8. Measure the extent of any scotoma. Place the stimulus in the scotoma (the location where static presentations were not seen). Now move the stimulus in a given direction until the patient reports that they can see it again. Mark this

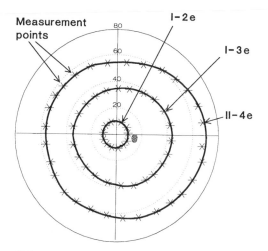

Fig. 10.1 *Measurement points connected together with an isopter line.*

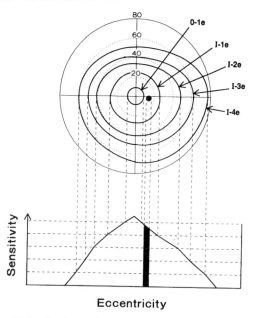

Fig. 10.2 *Static cut through the island of vision.*

location on the field chart. Move the stimulus back into the scotoma and move in a different direction until the stimulus is again seen. Repeat along different directions until a sufficient number of points have been located to accurately plot the extent of the scotoma. Note that when plotting the extent of a scotoma you always move from a non-seeing area to a seeing one. To measure the depth of a scotoma repeat the above with stimuli of different size and intensity. More accurate measures of scotoma depth can be obtained by profile perimetry (see below).

Profile perimetry

The Goldmann perimeter has an attachment that allows the perimetrist to determine the threshold at a series of points along a specified meridian. This type of examination is normally performed after a scotoma has been detected in an attempt to get more detailed information on its depth, the specified meridian being one that passes through a scotoma. This technique gives a static cut through the island of vision. The perimetrist first chooses the meridian and then a particular eccentricity along that meridian. The intensity of the stimulus is then gradually increased (1 dB steps, I-2d to I-2e is a 1 dB step) until the patient reports that they can see it. The chart (special charts are provided for static cuts, see Figure 10.2) is then marked with the appropriate intensity. The perimetrist then moves onto a neighbouring location, along the same meridian, and

repeats the procedure until a whole series of measurements are obtained. The points on the chart are then joined to give the static cut.

STATIC SUPRATHRESHOLD EXAMINATION (MULTIPLE STIMULUS)
Dicon perimeters, Fincham–Sutcliffe Screener, Friedmann Visual Field Analysers, Harrington Flocks Screener, Henson perimeters

This strategy is for rapid screening of the central field.

1. Train the patient. This can be done by first of all setting the stimulus intensity at a value well above the patient's threshold, i.e. at an intensity that they can easily see. Ask the patient to look at the fixation target and then present a stimulus pattern. All the above instruments are either manual or semi-automated and require the perimetrist to both select and present the stimulus patterns. Ask the patient how many lights they saw and then continue to present several other patterns, preferably with different numbers of stimuli, until you are happy that the patient understands the nature of the task.

2. Select the stimulus intensity. As the name implies, suprathreshold strategies are designed to

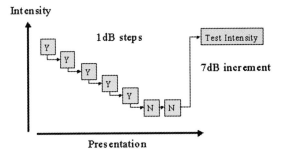

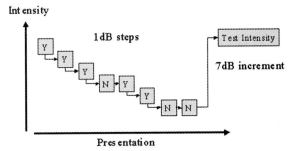

Fig. 10.3 *Technique for establishing the threshold at the onset of a threshold-related suprathreshold test.*

present their stimuli at an intensity that is above that of the patient's threshold. This intensity can be based upon (i) an initial quick measurement of the threshold (threshold-related), (ii) the patient's age (age-related), or (iii) fixed at some predetermined level (fixed intensity). The most accurate and most widely used technique is the threshold-related one.

3. Technique:
   (i) Threshold-related technique. This procedure can be used with all manual and semi-automated static instruments that have calibrated stimulus intensity scales, such as the Friedmann Analysers and Henson perimeters. The latest Henson perimeters incorporate this routine as a semi-automated procedure with instructions provided on screen.
      (a) Start off above the patient's threshold, i.e. at an intensity that the patient can easily see. The technique is diagrammatically represented in Figure 10.3.
      (b) Tell the patient that you will be presenting a series of patterns that will be get-

ting dimmer and dimmer until they become so dim that the patient will not be able to see them.
      (c) Decrease, in a stepwise manner (1 dB steps), changing the stimuli positions after each presentation until the patient reports that they cannot see the stimulus/i. It is advisable to present more than one pattern at this intensity to ensure that the original miss/es were not simply due to the stimuli falling in scotoma. Clearly, the more you present, the more confident you can be. Seven to eight stimulus locations (two multiple stimulus patterns) should be viewed as the minimum. Because 2 dB rather than 1 dB steps are normally used with the Friedmann Analysers the intensity at which the stimuli are all missed may be 1 dB below the true value. The perimetrist should bear this in mind when evaluating the results.
      (d) Increase the intensity by 6 or 7 dB for suprathreshold testing.
   (ii) Age-related technique. This technique is faster than the threshold-related one but not so accurate and has largely been replaced by the threshold-related technique. Set the intensity according to the age of the patient. Tables giving the appropriate value are normally provided with the instrument.
   (iii) Fixed intensity technique. This technique is found in some of the older instruments such as the Harrington Flocks Screener. The suprathreshold test intensity is fixed by the instrument.

4. Present all the stimulus patterns repeating, at the same intensity, any pattern in which one or more stimuli were missed. If stimuli were missed on both occasions ask the patient to tell you where the stimuli they saw (if any) were. (It is often helpful to tell the patient to consider the screen as a clock face and give the hour positions of the seen stimuli.) Mark on the chart, or enter into the computer, the missed stimulus/i. When stimuli are missed in the extreme superior part of the field the perimetrist should check that this is not due to a droopy eyelid or to the correcting lens rim.

5. After all the stimuli have been presented return to any that have been marked as missed and present them at gradually increasing intensities, marking down or entering into the computer the intensity at which the stimuli were eventually, if at all, seen.

STATIC SUPRATHRESHOLD EXAMINATION (SINGLE STIMULUS)
Dicon perimeters, Henson perimeters, Humphrey Visual Field Analyzers, Octopus perimeters

These instruments incorporate fully automated test strategies. The task of the perimetrist is simply to set the machine up, and to align and instruct the patient.

1. Train/instruct the patient. These instruments all use a patient response button which the patient is instructed to press every time they see a stimulus. There is normally a little demonstration routine at the beginning of the program to familiarize the patient with the task. Make sure that you run this routine and that the patient is perfectly happy about the task before you start collecting any data. In some instruments the demonstration routine is automatically run at the beginning of the test.
2. Select the stimulus intensity. The fully automated instruments incorporate set routines for finding the threshold that cannot be modified by the operator. Details on how some of these operate can be found in a later section of this chapter.
3. Present the suprathreshold stimuli. Again this part of the test is fully automated. While, in theory, the perimetrist is no longer needed after the examination has started, in practice more reliable results are obtained when the perimetrist stays in the room monitoring the results and giving supportive comments to the patient.

STATIC THRESHOLD PERIMETRY
Dicon perimeters, Henson perimeters, Humphrey Visual Field Analyzers, Octopus perimeters and others

This type of perimetry is used to establish the extent of any visual field loss. It is mainly used on patients who are either known to have a defect or on those in whom a defect is suspected, e.g. in the fellow eye of a patient with established loss in one eye. All the instruments cited above use single stimulus techniques and are fully automated. The task of the perimetrist is as follows.

1. Set the machine up, i.e. select the appropriate strategy and enter any required data such as the patient's age, name etc.
2. Select an appropriate lens correction, see Table 5.1 on page 54.
3. Align the patient.
4. Instruct the patient about the nature of the task. This aspect is very important. The patient should be told that their task is to keep looking at the fixation point in the centre of the screen and to press the response button every time they see a light flash. The perimetrist should stress that not all the presentations will be seen and that there is no reason to become alarmed when several presentations in a row are not seen as this is perfectly normal. The patient should be told that if they are unsure about whether or not they saw the stimulus then they should not press the response button. The patients should also be instructed on how to temporarily halt the program when needing a break. This is normally achieved by holding down the patient's response button.
5. Run the program. Instructions are normally given on the perimetrist's monitor.

ESTABLISHING THE THRESHOLD PRIOR TO A THRESHOLD-RELATED SUPRATHRESHOLD STRATEGY
At the beginning of a threshold-related suprathreshold strategy it is necessary for the perimetrist, or in the fully automated perimeters the perimeter, to get an estimate of the patient's threshold prior to setting the suprathreshold test intensity. The way this is done varies from one instrument to another. In the Humphrey Visual Field Analyzers the initial threshold estimate is automatically obtained from a measurement of the threshold at four retinal locations, one in each quadrant. At each location the threshold is measured with a two reversal bracketing

strategy (the technique used in their full-threshold strategy). It then uses the second most sensitive location to derive the hill of vision for the whole field and then tests at 6 dB above this (Humphrey, 1986). The remote chance of all four test locations falling within defective regions of the visual field is partly compensated for by not allowing the stimuli to go above a predetermined value. This technique is not very accurate. Henson *et al.*, (1999) reported that the precision of this technique was similar to that of the age-related technique when used on patient's without any field loss at the four seed locations and considerably worse than the age-related technique when there was some visual field loss at these locations.

Other researchers/instruments have recommended or adopted different techniques. For example, Batko *et al.* (1983), when conducting research with the Friedmann Visual Field Analyser, chose to use 'the weakest stimulus that could be seen at least one half of the time' and Gutteridge (1983), again with the Friedmann Visual Field Analyser, suggested using paracentral stimuli and decreasing their intensity until half or more escaped detection.

Henson and Anderson (1991) compared the accuracy of a series of different multiple stimulus techniques on a population of normal patients and concluded that a simple staircase technique, passing either from seeing to non-seeing or from non-seeing to seeing, gave a good compromise between accuracy and speed.

An important parameter in deciding which technique to use is its performance in the presence of visual field defects. What would happen to the threshold estimate if the patient had a hemianopia? Would they ever see more than 50% of the stimuli? Clearly, if we were to choose a criterion where the patient must see 50% of the presented stimuli, then the existence of this type of defect could lead to a considerable error, if indeed a threshold estimate could ever be established.

Henson and Anderson (1991) investigated this problem with a computer simulation. They found that one of the most robust techniques to the presence of a defect was to start off at an intensity below threshold and then increase it, in a stepwise manner, until one or more, out of a pattern of either three or four stimuli, were seen. Unfortunately, while this technique might be robust to the existence of a defect it is not patient-friendly. Presenting patterns of stimuli that are below the patient's threshold and continually asking them if they can see anything promotes uneasiness in the patient and with it the dangers of guessing. On the other hand, the technique of reducing the intensity, again in a stepwise manner, until a level is found at which none of the stimuli can be seen promotes patient well-being. The patient feels they are doing the right thing because they can see the stimuli, can see that the stimuli are getting dimmer and can recognize that soon they will not be able to see them, just indeed as the patient was told at the onset of the test. This type of threshold estimate also helps to train the patient. The results from this research led to the development of a new recommended technique for establishing the threshold prior to a threshold-related suprathreshold strategy. (see pp. 140–141).

REFERENCES

Batko K.A., Anctil J. and Anderson D.R. (1983) Detecting glaucomatous damage with the Friedmann Analyser compared with the Goldmann perimeter and evaluation of stereoscopic photographs of the optic disk. *Am J Ophthalmol*, **95**, 435–447.

Gutteridge IF. (1983) The working threshold approach to Friedmann visual field analyser screening. *Ophthalmic Physiol Optics*, **3**, 41–46.

Henson D.B. (1982) A proposed modification to the Fincham–Sutcliffe Screener. *Optician*, **183**, 4744 (June), 10–13.

Henson D.B. and Anderson R. (1991) Threshold-related suprathreshold field testing: which is the best technique of establishing the threshold? In *Perimetry Update 1990/91* (eds Mills R.P. and Heijl A.). Kugler & Ghedini, Amsterdam, pp. 367–372.

Henson D.B., Artes P.H., Chaudry S.J. and Chauhan B.C. (1999) Suprathreshold perimetry: establishing the test intensity. In *Perimetry Update 1998/1999* (eds Wall M. and Wild J.M.). Kugler & Ghedini, Amsterdam pp. 243–252.

Humphrey (1986) *The Field Analyzer Primer*. Allergan Humphrey, San Leandro, USA.

11 Visual field instruments

INTRODUCTION

It is always dangerous to put details concerning the specifications of instruments in a text such as this. No sooner has the text gone to press than a manufacturer changes the specifications of their instrument. Not to include such information would, however, be a disservice to the reader. Many readers want to know what the differences between instruments are without wading through piles of literature and review papers. It is for this reason that this chapter has attempted to bring together, in a consistent style, the specifications of many of the current generation of perimetric instruments. The Web site addresses are given for many of the instruments and these can be consulted for up-to-date information.

Several of the instruments described in this chapter are highly sophisticated, offering many different options to the perimetrist. These instruments are invariably computer controlled and are continually being re-programmed to give additional test strategies. Fortunately, most of the test strategies fall into one of a few different categories such as full-threshold or suprathreshold and differ only in the number and location of the test stimuli. This chapter will list the different strategies incorporated in each instrument; for further details on these the reader is referred to Chapter 3.

There is also insufficient space to give details on every piece of equipment that has ever been made. This chapter will, therefore, concentrate on those that, for one reason or another, have gained a degree of popularity.

The instruments are presented in alphabetical order.

BJERRUM SCREEN

Type. Flat field, central 25 degrees.

Target distance. 100 cm (200 cm versions are occasionally found).

Background luminance. Screen is black, illumination is normally set at 7 ft candles, although no facilities (or equipment) are provided to help set this value.

Stimuli. A series of white, red, green and blue painted discs ranging from 1 mm to 10 mm in diameter.

Description. The Bjerrum screen is a black cloth with a white fixation point attached at the centre. Black thread is sewn onto the screen in a series of radial and circumferential lines that are used to establish target position during the test.

In use one of the targets is attached to the end of a black wand which the perimetrist moves in from the periphery until seen by the patient. Scotoma within the area of an isopter are detected by continuing to move the target in towards the fixation point and asking the patient to report if, at any time, the target disappears. Black pins can be inserted into the cloth at the positions where the target appears/disappears. At the end of the test these positions are transferred to a field chart.

The main advantages of the Bjerrum screen are that it is cheap and versatile. It is possible to use a whole variety of different targets and to move them in any direction at whatever speed the perimetrist believes optimal.

Strategy. Kinetic.

Fixation. By direct observation of the patient.

Print out/storage of results. Results are manually drawn onto pre-printed chart paper.

Analysis of results. By visual inspection.

DICON TKS 5000, LD 400 AND SST AUTOPERIMETERS
Web page: http://dicon.com

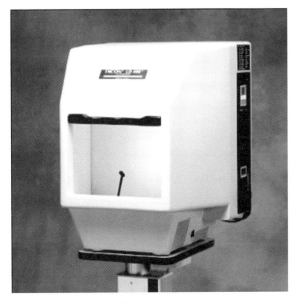

Fig. 11.1 *Dicon LD400.*

Type. Flat screen.

Target distance. 33.33 cm.

Background luminance. 10 cd/m^2 (31.5 asb).

Stimuli. Size – Goldmann IV, approximately 1 degree; LED peak emission – 565 nm; maximum intensity – 5000 asb; intensity steps – 1 dB; range – 50 dB; presentation time – 250 ms.

Description. Dicon produce a range of perimeters that use a movable fixation target to overcome the eccentricity limitations normally imposed by flat screens. The Dicon TKS is capable of presenting stimuli out to an eccentricity of 90 degrees while the LD (see Figure 11.1) and SST are capable of presenting stimuli out to an eccentricity of up to 60 degrees. The SST is a screening-only version of the LD 400 with a reduced number of test patterns (currently 6 versus 13).

The TKS and LD perimeters incorporate a voice synthesizer, which speaks to the patient (27 languages are currently available), providing instruction, encouragement and correction of errors. The patient can respond either with a conventional response button or verbally. Verbal responses ('zero, one, two, three, four') are interpreted by a voice recognition system.

Strategies. The Dicon instruments incorporate two test strategies: threshold-related suprathreshold and threshold. The threshold-related suprathreshold (5 dB above the threshold estimate) strategy can use single or multiple stimulus presentations and can be run with or without quantification, which takes the form of a threshold measurement of each missed point. The threshold strategy uses a 6–3 bracketing strategy and single stimulus presentations.

The current standard programs test from 40 to 80 locations in the central 30 degree field, 48 locations in the central 10 degrees, and from 72 to 120 locations in the full field (stimulus extend out to 60 degrees in the temporal field). In most programs the stimuli are arranged circumferentially, with one 30-2 grid pattern (6 degree square matrix offset by 3 degrees from the vertical and horizontal midlines covering the central 30 degrees), and a hybrid radial/grid pattern for glaucoma monitoring. Screening exams can be performed in either single or multiple stimulus presentations.

Fixation. Fixation is sampled with a Heijl–Krakau technique. All systems also report on the number of false positives and false negatives.

Printout/storage of results. TKS 5000, LD 400 and SST systems print data and grey scale results on an inkjet printer. Data can also be stored to disk or transferred (via serial port) to the 'FieldView' software package (TKS 5000, LD 400 only).

Analysis of results. Instrument printouts provide defect values. FieldView Omega (for DOS) and Advanced FieldView (for Windows) outputs provide further analysis including pointwise, global, quadrant and hemifield deviations based on either age or Relative Hill corrected data (this takes into account overall shifts in sensitivity values and is similar to pattern deviation values on the Humphrey Visual Field Analyzer). Probability maps are also presented indicating individual test locations that are significantly different from normal. Numeric and symbolic displays and grey scale overlays are colour-coded based on significance. Other analyses include 3-D Hill of Vision, Ranked Order, Meridional Profile, Isopter, and paired exam delta comparisons.

Advanced FieldView also offers multiple field displays and analysis of change over time.

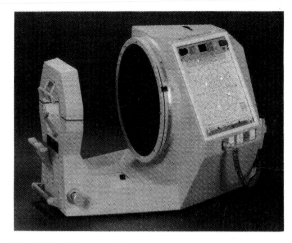

Fig. 11.2 *Friedmann Mark II Visual Field Analyser.*

FRIEDMANN VISUAL FIELD ANALYSER MARK I AND MARK II

Type. Flat field, central 25 degrees.

Target distance. 33 cm.

Background luminance. 0.1 cd/m^2

Stimuli. Number – 46(Mark I), 98(Mark II); type – white from a zenon discharge tube; size – varies with eccentricity; presentation time – approximately 0.5 msec.

Description. Both Friedmann Visual Field Analysers have been designed for quick routine screening of the visual field although the larger number of stimuli in the Mark II (see Figure 11.2) version gives it the facility to accurately mark out the extent of any defect. The Friedmann Visual Field Analysers present multiple stimulus patterns composed of either 2, 3 or 4 stimuli. These patterns are selected by the mechanical rotation of a fenestrated plate situated behind a second, stationary fenestrated plate. Light will only pass through these two plates when the fenestrations coincide. The light source is a single zenon discharge tube placed within an integrating bowl, the front of which is occluded by the fenestrated plates.

Patients verbally respond to each presentation, stating how many stimuli they saw.

The intensity of the stimuli can be altered by placing ND filters in front of the light source. These give a range of approx. 20 dB in 2 dB steps (1 dB steps are possible with the Mark II instrument but the mechanism for this has not been designed for routine use).

Defect depth can be measured by re-presenting missed stimuli at higher intensities.

Strategy/ies. The Friedmann Analysers use an eccentrically compensated (the stimulus size increases towards the periphery), multiple stimulus, suprathreshold strategy.

The initial threshold estimate is normally derived by measurement, i.e. threshold-related, although when originally developed in the late 1960s, it was intended to be used with an age-related strategy. Baseline information on the average threshold for each age group is provided with the instrument. As Friedmann instruments age their stimuli gradually get dimmer, which means that any age setting gradually becomes more and more inappropriate. The simplest solution to this problem, which cannot be overcome by replacing the bulb, is to use the more reliable threshold-related technique.

Fixation. By direct observation.

Print out/storage of results. Results are manually marked onto a pre-printed chart, which on the Mark II can be attached to the side of the instrument. There are no facilities for the storage of results.

Analysis of results. Analysis is by visual inspection.

GOLDMANN BOWL PERIMETER
Web page: http://www.haag-streit.com

Type. Bowl.

Target distance. 30 cm

Background luminance. $10 \, cd/m^2$ (31.5 asb).

Stimuli. The Goldmann stimuli are projected onto the inside surface of the bowl, which is painted white and has a coefficient of reflection of 0.7.

The standard Goldmann instrument has six different sizes of stimuli which are represented by the Roman numerals 0, I, II, III, IV and V. The size and angular subtence of these stimuli are given in Table 11.1.

Table 11.1 Size of stimuli used by Goldman

Goldmann size	Nominal size (mm^2)	Angular subtence (min of arc)
0	0.0625	3.78
I	0.25	7.68
II	1.0	15.36
III	4.0	30.71
IV	16	61.3
V	64	122.56

The original instrument had four stimulus intensities represented by the numbers 1 to 4, 4 being the brightest at 1000 asb. Intensities 3, 2 and 1 were obtained by placing 0.5, 1.0 and 1.5 log unit filters in front of the illuminating beam. In order to give a finer control of the stimulus intensity a second set of filters were later added, these being represented by the letters 'a' to 'e' and corresponding to 0.4, 0.3, 0.2, 0.1 and 0.0 log units. With a combination of the two sets of filters it is possible to change the intensity of the stimulus in 0.1 log unit steps over a range of 1.9 log units. Table 11.2 gives the stimulus intensities for each of the filter combinations.

It is also possible with the later Goldmann instruments to insert an additional 2.0 log unit filter to further extend the range of stimulus intensities to 5.9 log units. It is conventional to represent the presence of this filter by placing a bar over the filter number, e.g.

$\overline{2}e$ is a 3.0 log unit filter which attenuates to 1.0 asb.

The complete specification of a Goldmann stimulus is normally given with the size preceding the intensity given as a filter combination, e.g.

II-3e denotes stimulus size 'II', with filters '3' and 'e'.

While most perimetrists have learnt to use this system of stimulus specification, the more intuitive dB scale, used in most modern perimeters, would aid comprehension for the newcomer.

Description. The Goldmann perimeter is a manual bowl perimeter capable of presenting its stimuli out to an eccentricity of 90 degrees. It uses a pantographic arrangement to connect the stimulus projector to a stylus held by the perimetrist over the visual field chart. The position of the stimulus, within the

Table 11.2 Log attenuation and stimulus intensity of the Goldmann instrument

Filter	Log units	Intensity (asb)	Intensity (cd/m^2)
4e	0.0	1000	318.0
4d	0.1	800	255.0
4c	0.2	630	200.0
4b	0.3	500	160.0
4a	0.4	400	127.0
3e	0.5	320	102.0
3d	0.6	250	80.0
3c	0.7	200	64.0
3b	0.8	160	51.0
3a	0.9	130	41.0
2e	1.0	100	31.8
2d2	1.1	80	25.5
2c	1.2	63	20.1
2b	1.3	50	15.9
2a	1.4	40	12.7
1e	1.5	32	10.2
1d	1.6	25	8.0
1c	1.7	20	6.4
1b	1.8	16	5.1
1a	1.9	13	4.1

patient's field, corresponds to the location of the stylus on the field chart. This system is extremely flexible, the perimetrist can move the stylus, and hence the stimulus, in whatever direction and at whatever speed he or she wishes.

The Goldmann perimeter is often used as a standard to which other perimeters are compared and can be found in practically every department of ophthalmology. It is extremely versatile and can be used to examine either the central or peripheral field.

The selected stimulus is normally continuously on, although there is a facility to either briefly present or extinguish it with the aid of a manually controlled shutter. It is not possible to accurately control presentation time.

Strategy. The Goldmann perimeter was designed to use kinetic strategies, although it is often used in a pseudo static mode to spot check certain locations, e.g. Armaly Drance routine. It can also be fitted with an attachment that allows it to produce static cuts across the visual field.

Fixation. By direct observation with the aid of a telescope.

Printout/storage of results. Results are manually drawn onto pre-printed chart paper. There are no facilities for the electronic storage of data.

Analysis of results. By visual inspection.

HENSON PERIMETERS
Web page: http://www.henson-vfa.com

Tinsley Medical Instruments currently manufacture two perimeters, the Henson CFA3200 (earlier versions of which were called the Henson CFS2000 and Henson CFA3000) and the Henson Pro (earlier version Henson 4000). The main difference between these two instruments is that the Henson Pro is a bowl perimeter capable of testing out to an eccentricity of 72 degrees while the CFA3200 is a flat screen central field analyser capable of testing out to an eccentricity of 25 degrees.

The current range of Henson instruments use a series of graded examination strategies. In the supra-threshold strategies these start off with just 26 test points. This examination is designed to be used on patients in whom there is no suspicion of a visual field defect, i.e. for screening purposes. The second level increases the number of test locations to 68. It is designed for patients in whom there is some suspicion, either as a result of them missing one or more of the screening stimuli or because of some other parameter such as raised IOP. The third level increases the number of locations to 136. It is designed to be used when the clinician wishes to evaluate the extent of a defect. These three levels can be run one after the other. If at the end of one level the perimetrist wishes to test more locations then the test is simply extended. The graded approach is also used in threshold testing, e.g. the operator can start off with a 24-2 program and extend it to a 30-2 should clinical need arise.

All current Henson instruments also allow the operator to re-test and/or delete any test location and to add new test locations. This facility allows the perimetrist to remove/correct artefactual data, such as that arising from lid artefacts. It also allows the perimetrist to increase the number of test locations in and around a suspect/defect region.

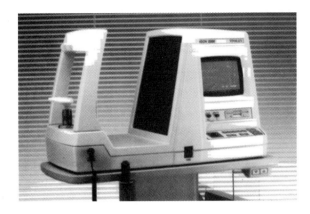

Fig. 11.3 *Henson 3200.*

Henson CFA3200 (early versions CFS2000 and CFA3000)

Type. Flat screen.

Target distance. 33 cm.

Background luminance. 0.25 cd/m^2.

Stimuli. Number – 220; type – LED with broad spectral output (530–600 nm); maximum intensity – 300 cd/m^2; intensity step – 1 dB.; size – 0.5 degrees; presentation time – 200 msec.

Description. The Henson CFS2000 was first launched in 1985 and replaced by the CFA3000, in 1989. The main difference between the CFA3000 and the CFS2000 is that the CFA3000 incorporates a full-threshold program (see below for more details). The CFA3000 was replaced by the CFA3200 in 1995 (see Figure 11.3). The 3200 incorporated a larger number of stimuli with options to present these one at a time in order to validate findings from pre-programmed test patterns.

These instruments use LED stimuli that have flat, diffusing front surfaces and are flush mounted within a flat grey screen. The reflective properties of the screen are matched to that of the LEDs (when they are off), thereby minimizing any black hole effect.

A monitor, attached to the side of the instrument, relays the current status of the selected program and the results of the examination as it proceeds. Operator interaction is via small keyboard.

Strategy/ies. All instruments incorporate a multiple stimulus (two to four stimuli per presentation) suprathreshold strategy, which is eccentrically compensated and designed to be used in the threshold-related manner. The suprathreshold increment is set at 5 dB above the threshold estimate and there is a facility for quantifying defect depth by using 8 and 12 dB suprathreshold increments.

The suprathreshold test uses the graded approach described above. The full-threshold program of the CFA3000/3200 tests 52 locations (6 degree matrix offset 3 degrees from the vertical and horizontal midlines) within the central 25 degrees of the visual field. It uses a repetitive bracketing strategy with step sizes of 4 dB reducing to 2 dB after the first reversal.

Catch trials are incorporated in the single stimulus strategies to estimate false positive and false negative response rates.

Fixation. Fixation monitoring in the suprathreshold strategies is by direct observation and in the full-threshold strategy by the Heijl–Krakau technique.

Print out/storage of results. The results from both strategies are printed out with grey scale symbols representing the depth of any defect. The print out from the full-threshold strategy also includes numeric data.

Analysis of results. All models incorporate software that analyses the results of the suprathreshold program and gives an indication of the likelihood that the current response comes from a normal patient. This result, which includes a cluster analysis routine (see Chapter 9 on quantification) are displayed on a scale divided into 'normal', 'suspect' and 'defect'.

The full-threshold program of the CFA3000/3200 calculates the global indices mean defect, loss variance, corrected loss variance and fluctuation.

Henson Pro

Type. Bowl.

Target distance. 25 cm.

Background luminance. 3.15 cd/m^2, 10 asb.

Stimuli. LEDs with broad spectral output (530–600 nm) back-projected onto diffusing surface;

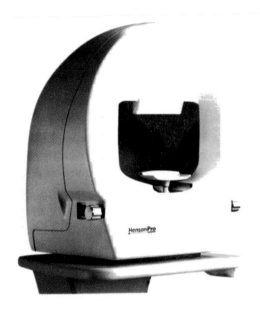

Fig. 11.4 *Henson Pro.*

maximum intensity – 1000 cd/m² with a range of 48 dB; intensity steps – 1 dB; size – 0.5 degrees.; presentation time – 200 ms.

Description. The Henson Pro (see Figure 11.4) is a compact bowl perimeter which can be mounted on a standard instrument table. The perimeter is controlled via an IBM PC which is either incorporated into the instrument (Pro 3500) or separated (Pro 5000). The PC monitor gives the present status of the examination as well as giving a range of options through a series of pull-down menus. Data can be input either via a touch screen, pointing device (mouse, trackerball, touchpad etc.) or a separate QWERTY keyboard. A separate monitor relays an image of the patient's eye from a built-in CCD camera. The software operates through the Microsoft Windows environment and incorporates a Windows Help facility.

The Henson Pro can present stimuli on a 3 degree square matrix within the central 30 degrees of the field and a 6 degree square matrix in the peripheral field. The position of the fixation light occasionally changes when examining the peripheral field.

Strategy/ies. The Henson Pro offers a large range of single and multiple stimulus suprathreshold strategies. Some of these are designed to operate over the central 25 degrees of the visual field while others test out to an

eccentricity of 72 degrees. All suprathreshold strategies utilize the graded approach described above. The Henson Pro also includes two fixed intensity tests for vehicle drivers, one based on the Esterman distribution of stimuli and the other specifically designed to meet the UK driver's test visual field requirements.

The Henson Pro incorporates two threshold strategies, full-threshold (two reversal, 4 dB steps reducing to 2 dB after the first reversal) and fast-threshold (one reversal, 3 dB steps). There are a large number of stimulus distributions covering the central, peripheral and macular regions. Catch trials are incorporated in the single stimulus strategies to estimate both false positive and false negative response rates.

Fixation. Fixation is monitored with both the Heijl–Krakau technique (full-threshold tests) and a CCD video camera that relays an image of the patient's eye to a dedicated monitor.

Printout/storage of results. Results are printed out in both grey scale and numeric format. Results can be stored for later recall/analysis in a Windows-based database.

Analysis of results. Suprathreshold strategies are analysed in the same way as the CFA3200, giving an estimate of the likelihood of the result coming from a normal patient. Threshold examinations calculate the indices, mean defect, loss variance, corrected loss variance and fluctuation. Pattern deviation probability values are also given for central full-threshold tests.

Data from suprathreshold and threshold tests can be serially analysed within the database. This takes the form of multiple displays and graphical plots of global indices (threshold tests) and number of missed locations (suprathreshold tests).

HUMPHREY VISUAL FIELD ANALYZERS
Web page: http://www.humphrey.com
http://www.peridata.org
http://www.obflabs.com

Zeiss instruments currently manufacture the 700 series of the Humphrey Visual Field Analyzer. The 700 series took over from the 600 series in 1994. The 700 series is more compact and includes some additional test strategies. Within each series there are a variety of models which outwardly appear the same

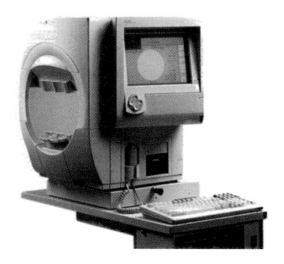

Fig. 11.5 *Humphrey Visual Field Analyzer (700 series).*

and use the same mechanism to present the stimuli and to record the patient's responses. The differences between the models include the number and type of programs, the addition of a video camera to help monitor fixation, the type and size of the storage devices and facilities such as blue–yellow perimetry and advanced statistical analysis of the data.

700 series Humphrey Visual Field Analyzers

Type. Bowl.

Target distance. 33 cm at the fixation point reducing towards the periphery in order to keep the size of the instrument small.

Background luminance. $10 \, \text{cd/m}^2$.

Stimuli. Type – projection; maximum intensity – $3183 \, \text{cd/m}^2$; intensity step – 1 dB; size – Goldmann I–V; presentation time – 200 msec.

Description. The Humphrey Visual Field Analyzer (see Figure 11.5) is a bowl perimeter which projects its stimuli onto the inside surface of the bowl. A monitor, on the side of the instrument, presents a series of menus at the beginning of the test. Operator interaction is via a light pen/touch screen. The 700 series can also be controlled via a QWERTY keyboard.

Strategy/ies. The Humphrey instrument offers a large range of single stimulus, threshold-related and age-related suprathreshold strategies. They differ in the number and location of the stimuli, whether they quantify the results from missed stimuli, and the nature of any quantification.

The 700 series incorporate three threshold strategies, full-threshold (two reversal, 4 dB steps reducing to 2 dB after the first reversal) fast-threshold (one reversal, 3 dB steps) and SITA (see Chapter 3, pp. 36, 37). There is a range of test patterns for each strategy, including central, peripheral and macular. Catch trials are incorporated to estimate false positive and false negative response rates in the full- and fast-threshold strategies. In the SITA strategy false positive catch trials are replaced by an analysis of response times.

Fixation. Fixation is monitored with the Heijl–Krakau technique and, on the more expensive models, with a video camera which relays its image to the monitor.

Print out/storage of results. Results are printed out in a variety of forms, including grey scale, numeric and profile formats. In addition to this, the results can be stored on a built-in disk drive for later recall/analysis.

Analysis of results. A software package, STATPAC, analyses the results from the threshold programs. This package calculates the indices, mean deviation, pattern standard deviation, fluctuation and corrected pattern standard deviation. It also produces a probability map indicating individual test locations that are significantly different from normal.

The STATPAC package also incorporates facilities for serial analysis of visual field data including a pointwise change analysis and a global regression analysis.

The Humphrey instruments do not analyse the results from suprathreshold programs.

Analysis of Humphrey visual field data can also be performed within the software packages PeriData and Progressor. For more information on these see the Web pages given above.

OCTOPUS PERIMETERS

Web page: http://www.interzeag.haag-streit.com
http://www.peridata.org

Interzeag currently manufacture two different Octopus

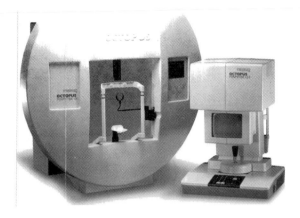

Fig. 11.6   *Octopus perimeters 101 and 1-2-3.*

perimeters. There is the Octopus 1-2-3, which is a compact office perimeter, testing out to an eccentricity of 30 degrees, and the Octopus 101, a bowl perimeter that tests out to an eccentricity of 90 degrees. Earlier models include the pioneering 201 developed in 1976, the 2000 and 500.

Octopus 1-2-3

Type. Direct projection (see below) central 30 degrees.

Target distance. Targets are optically placed at infinity.

Background luminance. $10\,cd/m^2$ $(31.4\,asb)$.

Stimuli. Type – LED with broad spectral output 560–670 nm; maximum intensity – $1273\,cd/m^2$ (4000 asb); intensity steps – 1 dB; size – Goldmann III and V; presentation time – 100, 200 or 500 msec.

Description. The Octopus 1-2-3 (see Figure 11.6) uses a system called direct projection in which the stimuli are imaged at infinity with a large aperture lens placed just in front of the patient's spectacle plane. This system removes the need for a cupola or screen and thereby reduces the overall size of the instrument. It also makes the instrument relatively independent of ambient lighting.

A monitor attached to the back of the instrument presents the operator with a series of menus at the beginning of the test and current status of the test

during the examination. The output of the fixation-monitoring camera can also be viewed on the monitor.

Strategy/ies. The instrument incorporates four different testing strategies: suprathreshold screening (testing at 4 dB above the age normative values), full-threshold (two reversal, 4 dB steps reducing to 2 dB after the first reversal), dynamic threshold and Tendency Orientated Perimetry (TOP) (see Chapter 3). All of the programs are divided into a series of different stages (see below).

There are a number of different stimulus patterns, including ones specifically for glaucoma, the macular and general examinations. There is also a facility for the user to write custom test programs for the central 30 degrees.

The 1-2-3 uses a graded approach to visual field testing (staging). Test programs are broken down into different phases with extensions allowing (a) the quantification of relative defects, (b) repeat quantitative testing and (c) extension of the test area. The decision on whether or not to complete each stage does not have to be made until the end of the preceding stage, i.e. the testing can be customized to the nature of the results obtained during the early stages of the examination. This facility is similar to the extend facility on the Henson perimeters.

Catch trials are incorporated to estimate false positive and false negative response rates.

Fixation. The Octopus 1-2-3 incorporates an automatic monitoring system which checks the amount of light reflected from the pupillary region prior to each stimulus presentation. If this does not fall within accepted limits then it is assumed that fixation has been lost and the data rejected (see Chapter 5, p. 57).

The image from the video camera can also be viewed on the operator's monitor for direct observation.

Printout/storage of results. Results are printed out in a variety of different formats, including grey scale, numeric, defect, probability and Bebie curve (see Chapter 9, p. 126). Data can be stored on a separate computer system connected to the perimeter.

Analysis of results. Global indices, mean defect, loss variance, corrected loss variance and fluctuation are derived from the threshold strategies (full, dynamic and TOP). Two of these indices (mean defect and loss variance) are continuously calculated and displayed throughout the test rather than waiting until the whole examination is finished.

The software incorporates a 'Defect level indicator', which graphically displays the current mean defect value along with its confidence limits on a scale that goes from 'normal' to 'depressed'. By looking at this indicator the perimetrist can rapidly decide whether or not further testing is needed.

When connected to a separate computer (IBM PC), two computer programs, PeriTrend and PeriData, can be used for the storage and later recall and analysis of visual field data (see web pages, given at the beginning of this section, for more detail). These programs also offer a wider range of printout formats and facilities for comparing visual fields and plotting trends. Several perimeters can be connected to the same computer.

Octopus 101

Type. Bowl.

Target distance. 42.5 cm.

Background luminance. Standard 4 asb but can be set to 0, 31.4 or 314 asb. (314 used for blue–yellow perimetry.)

Stimuli. Type – projection; maximum intensity – 1000 asb; intensity steps – 1 dB over a 40 dB range; size – Goldmann 1–V; presentation time – 100, 200 or 500 msec.

Description. The Octopus 101 (see Figure 11.6) is a bowl perimeter controlled by a separate computer (IBM PC) operating through Microsoft Windows environment. A single computer can control a number of different perimeters. It is basically a static perimeter but can also perform kinetic and blue–yellow perimetry.

Strategy/ies. The 101 offers the same four static test strategies as the 1-2-3, i.e. suprathreshold screening, full-threshold, dynamic and TOP (see above for more details).

The kinetic strategy is provided largely for the testing of the peripheral field. The software incorporates a facility for displaying peripheral kinetic results and central static results on the same chart.

Because it is a bowl perimeter the 101 incorporates a larger range of test patterns, including glaucoma, macula and neurological. There is also a facility for the user to write custom test programs.

Catch trials are incorporated to estimate false positive and false negative response rates.

Fixation. The Octopus 101 incorporates a CCD camera that relays an image of the eye to the PC where it is displayed in the top left-hand corner of the monitor. It also contains an automatic fixation monitoring system.

Printout/storage of results. Results are printed out in a variety of different formats, including grey scale, numeric, defect, probability and Bebie curve (see Chapter 9, p. 125). The computer can store large amounts of data for subsequent recall and analysis.

Analysis of results. Global indices, mean defect, loss variance, corrected loss variance and fluctuation are derived from the threshold strategies (full, dynamic and TOP).

The 101 also includes the Defect level indicator described above.

PeriTrend and PeriData are two programs for the storage, printing and statistical analysis of Octopus data. PeriTrend has been specifically developed for the Octopus while PeriData is an independent software package that can also deal with the results from a selected range of other perimeters.

PeriTrend can display up to six examinations on a single screen. The mode of the display can be set to any of the common output formats, e.g. thresholds, Bebie curves, probability maps etc. This software can also plot the trends of the global indices, mean defect, loss variance and corrected loss variance and indicate whether or not there is a significant improvement or deterioration in the values.

PeriData has many of the functions described above for PeriTrend but has the additional facility of performing a pointwise linear regression analysis. The results from this analysis are presented in a variety of formats. One simply gives the computed start and end values for the series along with the significance level of any change. The GATT (Global Analysis of Topographical Trends) format gives a grey scale presentation in which horizontal lines indicate deterioration and vertical ones improvement. The GANT (Global Analysis of Numerical Trends) format gives a Bebie curve of the computed 'start' values along with vertical lines which represent the amount of change.

Glossary of terms

Age-related test
A suprathreshold test in which the intensity of the test stimuli are set according to the patient's age.

Amsler charts
A set of charts used for testing the central visual field. Also known as Amsler grids.

Angioscotoma
A scotoma produced by the retinal vessels passing in front of the receptors.

Apostilb, asb
A luminance unit of measurement.

Arcuate scotoma
A scotoma that arcs around the fixation point following the course of the retinal nerve fibres.

Candela per square metre, cd/m^2
A luminance unit of measurement.

Cecocentral
See Centrocecal.

Centrocecal
The area of retina that includes the macula, the optic nerve head and the area in between.

Confrontation test
A visual field screening test in which the perimetrist sits facing the patient.

Congenital crescents
See tilted optic disc

Congruous

A congruous field defect is one that affects the same region of the field of both eyes.

Contralateral

Opposite side.

Conus

See tilted optic disc

Decibel, dB

A unit of attenuation. 10 dB is equivalent to 1 log unit.

Eccentrically compensated

A suprathreshold test in which the test stimulus intensity is adjusted to compensate for the normal variations in sensitivity across the visual field.

Esterman grid

A method of scoring the extent of visual field. Different grids are available for the central field, whole field and binocular field. Used in litigation and more recently, in its binocular form, as a test for drivers.

False negative

The patient failed to respond to a stimulus presentation at an intensity estimated to be above their threshold.

False positive

The patient responded to a dummy stimulus presentation.

Fixed intensity test

The intensity of the stimuli is the same for all patients. No account is taken of how the sensitivity of the eye changes with age or of the variations that occur within any particular age group.

Fluctuation

Variability in the visual field. Often divided into 'short-term', that which occurs during a single visual field examination, and 'long-term', the additional component that is seen to exist between visual field examinations.

Frequency-of-seeing (FOS) curve

An S-shaped graph depicting the likelihood of seeing a stimulus over a range of intensities.

Fuch's coloboma

See tilted optic disc

Functional loss

Field loss due to an impairment of function rather than structure. Malingering and hysteria are forms of functional loss.

Glaucoma hemifield test (GHT)

A quantification technique that establishes whether or not a visual field result falls within the normal limits. It compares the threshold values in the superior visual hemifield to those in the inferior hemifield.

Global indices

Quantification values which represent the whole of the visual field.

Gradient-adapted

See eccentrically compensated.

Hemianopia

A field defect affecting one half of the visual field.

Homonymous

Affecting the same side.

Incongruous

The opposite of congruous.

Ipsilateral

Same side.

Isopter

A line that joins together points of equal sensitivity.

Kinetic perimetry

A form of perimetry in which the stimulus is moved.

Lens rim artefact

Scotoma caused by the rim of a correcting lens.

Long-term fluctuation

See Fluctuation

Macular sparing
When the central 5–10 degrees is unaffected in an otherwise hemianopic defect.

Mesopic
A range of intensity levels lying between the photopic and scotopic ranges.

Miosis
A reduced pupil size.

Multiple stimulus test
Stimuli are presented in patterns of 2, 3 or 4. The patient responds, usually verbally, by stating how many of the stimuli they saw.

One level test
In this form of test the stimuli are all presented at the same intensity. No account is taken of the fact that the eye's retinal sensitivity varies with eccentricity.

Papillomacular bundle
The bundle of nerve fibres arising from the macular.

Perimeter
An instrument designed for perimetry.

Perimetry
The study of the visual field.

Photopic
The range of intensity levels at which the eye is light-adapted.

Quadrantanopsia
Loss of a quadrant.

Reliability criteria
A term that collectively applies to false positive and false negative response errors along with fixation errors.

Scotoma
An isolated area of depressed or absent sensitivity.

Sensitivity
An index of test performance calculated as the percentage of patients correctly identified by the test.

Short-term fluctuation
See Fluctuation

Single stimulus
The stimuli are presented one at a time.

SITA (Swedish Interactive Thresholding Strategy)
Threshold strategy that utilizes prior information to reduce the number of presentations and duration of the examination.

Situs inversus
See tilted optic disc.

Specificity
An index of test performance calculated as the percentage of cases without field loss who are correctly classified as not having any visual field loss.

Static perimetry
A form of perimetry in which the locations of the stimuli are fixed.

Suprathreshold test
In this type of strategy stimuli are presented at an intensity which is calculated to be above the patient's threshold. If the stimulus is seen by the patient then it is assumed that no significant defect exists.

Tangent screen
A flat screen used for testing the central field.

Threshold test
A test strategy in which a measurement or estimate of the threshold is made at a whole series of predetermined retinal locations. Each estimate usually involves presenting a stimulus several times at each retinal location with a repetitive bracketing strategy.

Threshold-related test
A suprathreshold test in which the stimuli are presented at an intensity based upon a measured estimate of the patient's sensitivity made at the beginning of the examination.

Tilted optic disc
A congenital anomaly in which the optic disc appears tilted to the nasal rather than temporal side.

Index